THE COMPLETE ANTI-INFLAMMATORY COOKBOOK

50 Recipes to Protect You and Your Family From Inflammation and Heart Diseases

Artsy Chef

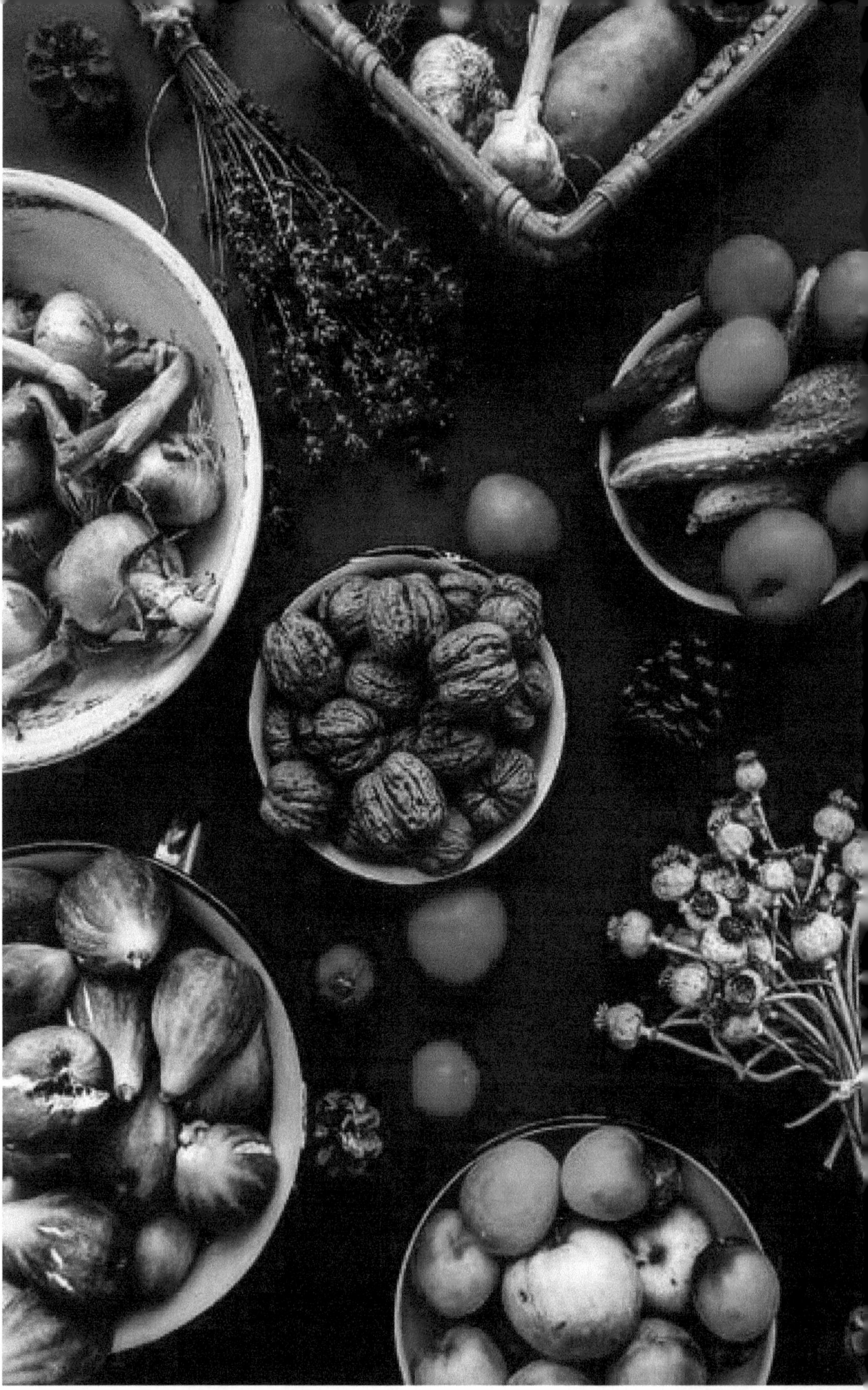

inattention, use, or misuse of the information in question by the reader will render any resulting actions solely under their purview. There are no scenarios in which the publisher or the original author of this work can be in any fashion deemed liable for any hardship or damages that may befall them after undertaking the information described herein.

Additionally, the information in the following pages is intended only for informational purposes and should thus be thought of as universal. As befitting its nature, it is presented without assurance regarding its prolonged validity or interim quality. Trademarks that are mentioned are done without written consent and can in no way be considered an endorsement from the trademark holder.

Table of Contents

INTRODUCTION 1

BREAKFAST 23

    Corn Bowl.. 24

    Lemon Tomatoes 26

    Blueberry Porridge 27

    Nutmeg Oats 28

    Pineapple Bowl 30

    Pumpkin Pie Spices Quinoa 31

    Nutmeg Pork 32

    Rosemary Pork Cubes............................. 34

LUNCH 35

    Cod and Tarragon Sauce........................ 37

    Orange Chicken Salad............................ 39

    Brown Rice with Chicken 41

    Greek Chicken Breasts............................ 43

    Easy Chicken with Potato 46

Paprika Chicken Mix.......................................48

Grilled Eggplant Salad 50

Eggplant with Avocado Lunch 52

Eggplant with Egg 55

SNACKS & APPETIZERS 57

Simple Peanut Butter Dip...........................59

Easy Nutmeg Apple Snack..........................60

Dill Coconut Dip 61

Sweet Potato and Sesame Spread 63

Dill Zucchini Patties....................................65

Simple Cauliflower Crackers.......................67

Baked Mushroom Caps 69

Almond Spinach Dip....................................71

DINNER 73

Baked Leek...74

Broccoli Steaks..75

Thyme Haddock 77

Nutmeg Trout 78

Cayenne Pepper Shrimps 80

Tomato Calamari... 81

Chicken and Beans 82

Chicken with Green Beans.................................. 84

Chicken and Beets 85

SOUPS 86

Sweet Soup 87

Parsnip Cream Soup 89

Wedges Soup 91

Curry Soup 93

Lentils Soup.. 94

Mushroom Cream Soup 95

Meatball Soup 97

Tropical Soup 98

DESSERTS 99

Pomegranate Bowls 101

Maple Berries Bowls.. 102

Almond Rhubarb Pudding 103

Dates and Pears Cake 105

Pears Cream..106

Orange Bowls..107

Chicory Cherry Cream 108

Cinnamon Apple Mix..110

INTRODUCTION

The anti-inflammatory diet is the best diet for conditions that cause inflammation such as asthma, chronic peptic ulcer, tuberculosis, rheumatoid arthritis, period on it is Crohn's disease, sinusitis, active hepatitis, etc. Along with medical treatment, proper nutrition is very important. An anti-inflammatory diet can help to reduce the pain from inflammation and supplement other treatments.

Inflammation is a natural response of your body to infections, injuries, and illnesses. The classic symptoms are redness, pain, heat, and swelling. Nevertheless, some diseases such as diabetes, heart disease, and cancer produce no symptoms. An anti-inflammatory diet is a great preventive way to safeguard your health.

The anti-inflammatory diet provides antioxidants and reduces the level of free radicals in our bodies. The most common question that people ask is what to eat while on the anti-inflammatory diet. Recommended foods are fruit, vegetables, whole grains, plant-based proteins, and fish, as well as spices, condiments, and dressings. The only condition that should be followed is that all food should be organic.

The most popular vegetables and fruits for the diet are leafy greens, cherries, raspberries, blackberries, tomatoes, cucumbers, etc. Grains include oatmeal, brown rice, and all grains that are high in fiber. Herbs and spices are natural antioxidants that will boost your health as they add flavor. You should avoid highly processed food such as sugary drinks, chocolate, ice cream, French fries, burgers, sausages, deli meats, and overly greasy food. One more factor that will help is making sure you get enough water per day. It is easy to track. There are a lot of apps that will help you to do it correctly. Drinking plenty of water helps the body to cleanse faster.

The anti-inflammatory diet is simple to follow and is not restrictive. There are many ways to adjust it to your preferences. Nevertheless, there are some cons that you should know. It can be costly since it recommends eating all organic food. It also contains a lot of allergens such as nuts, seeds, and soy.

However, eating the right adjusted food will help to eliminate the cons of the diet. It is highly recommended to go to your doctor for a complete medical examination before starting the diet.

This is important information that you should know before starting any diet. A diet is not a magic remedy for all diseases, but it does support the body in conjunction with treatment. Start your new healthy life with one small step, and you will see huge results within half a year. You can be sure that your body will respond by giving you a fresh look and energy for new achievements.

What to Eat and Avoid on the Anti-Inflammatory Diet

- **Meat, Poultry, and Fish**

The best choice for an anti-inflammatory diet is fish and seafood. This type of food is rich in omega-3 fatty acids. Meat can be eaten in moderation, although it is recommended to eat grass-fed meat.

What to eat	Eat occasionally	What to avoid
Tuna	Beef	Lamb
Sole	Chicken	Lard
Shrimps	Pork loin	Bacon
Turkey	Pork tenderloin	pork
Halibut		Breaded fish
Trout		
Salmon		
Flounder		

Mackerel		
Oysters		
Sardines		
Catfish		
Clams		
Cod		
Crab		
Herring		

- **Dairy**

Dairy products can be both useful and harmful to your health. Full-fat dairy products can cause acne and increase inflammatory conditions.

What to eat	Eat occasionally	What to avoid
Non-fat milk	Rice milk	Whole cream
Low-fat milk	Skim milk	Sour cream

Coconut milk	Tofu cheese	Cream
Greek-style yogurt	Parmesan	Hard cheese
		Milk butter
Fat-free plain traditional yogurt		Margarine
		Cottage cheese
Cashew butter		
Sunflower seeds butter		

- **Eggs**

Eggs contain essential nutrients, proteins, lutein, and zeaxanthin, which all fight inflammation. Nevertheless, frequent consumption of eggs can cause allergic reactions.

- **Nuts and Seeds**

Nuts and seeds are good for heart health. They are rich in fiber and nutrition. Only eat them if you're sure you have no sensitivities.

What to eat	Eat occasionally	What to avoid
Almonds	Hazelnuts	Chocolate-covered nuts
Chia seeds	Cashews	Nut butter (sweetened/ unsweetened)
Flaxseeds	Peanut butter	
Pumpkin seeds		Macadamia nuts
Pistachios		Peanuts
		Pecans

- **Vegetables**

The main source of vitamins during the anti-inflammatory diet is vegetables. However, not all vegetables are beneficial. Avoid starchy vegetables and vegetables that can cause allergic reactions.

What to eat	Eat occasionally	What to avoid
Sweet potatoes	Tomatoes	Potatoes
Yams	Tomatillos	Potato chips
Beets	Corn	Mushrooms
Radishes		
Watermelon		
Green beans		
Organic baked corn chips		
Sweet peppers		
Shiitake mushrooms		
Bell peppers		

- **Fruits and Berries**

Fruits are rich in vitamins. Nevertheless, avoid eating large amounts of sugary fruits. Replace them with sweet and sour or sour fruits/berries.

What to eat	Eat occasionally	What to avoid
Tart cherries	Kiwi	Acerola
Strawberries	Papaya	Lychee
Blueberries	Bananas	Persimmon
Apples		
Pears		
Apricots		
Avocado		
Dried fruits		

Oranges		
Mangoes		
Pineapple		

- **Grain Products**

Whole-grains are rich in fiber and can fight inflammation and protect our body from infection. Avoid eating "bad" grains.

What to eat	What to avoid
Brown rice	White rice
Wild rice	Sugar cereals
Oatmeal	White bread
Whole-grain bread	Crackers
Multigrain bread	Snacks
Whole-grain pasta	Rye bread
Oat flour	Wheat noodles
Buckwheat flour	White bread crumbs
Whole wheat flour	Corn flour

Rice noodles	Wheat tortillas
Corn tortillas	Bagels
Whole-grain toast	

- **Condiments**

Condiments play a significant role in flavor. They can make a meal tender, spicy, or salty. On your anti-inflammatory diet, you can use almost all spices and herbs. They have strong anti-inflammatory features.

What to eat	What to avoid
Low-fat mayonnaise	Mayonnaise (full-fat)
Ground pink peppercorns	Tartar sauce
Turmeric tahini dressing	Teriyaki
Alfredo sauce	Tomato sauce
Hot red pepper sauce	Bordelaise sauce
Chimichurri sauce	Brown sauce
Curry powder	Chili sauce
Tapatio sauce (handmade)	Dijon sauce
Apple cider vinegar	Buffalo sauce
	Hollandaise sauce

Pomegranate sauce	Marinara sauce
	Worcestershire sauce
	Sweet and sour sauce
	Soy sauce
	Pickle relish
	Barbecue sauce
	Dijon mustard

- **Oils and fats**

It is recommended to consume vegetable oils and fats during the anti-inflammatory diet. Bear in mind that some natural oils can cause allergies.

What to eat	Eat occasionally	What to avoid
Sunflower oil (cold-pressed) Grapes seed oil	Walnut oil	Coconut oil Palm oil

Olive oil (extra virgin)		
Flax seeds oil		

- **Beverages**

Drinking water should be a rule for you during the anti-inflammatory diet. Nevertheless, not all drinks are created equal. Avoid consuming sparkling drinks and beverages that contain artificial sugars.

What to eat	Eat occasionally	What to avoid
Fresh fruits	Fresh juice	Coffee
Seltzer		Sodas
Filtered water		Wine
Mineral water		Sparkling mineral water
Lemon water		Carbonated drinks
Herbal tea		Sweet sparkling beverages

Green tea		
Mate tea		

- **Sweets**

Fruits are the best sweets during the anti-inflammatory diet. They are rich in vitamins and contain only natural sweeteners.

Nevertheless, you can find a lot of sugar-free meals which are not inferior in taste to the most famous desserts.

What to eat	Eat occasionally	What to avoid
Honey	Stevia	Artificial sweeteners
Raw cocoa powder	Xylitol	Buns
Fruits (allowed for anti-inflammatory diet)	Brown rice syrup	Candy
	Dark chocolate	Cakes
		Chocolate
		Cookies

		Custard
		Ice cream
		Pastries
		Pies
		Pudding
		Sugar
		Tarts
		Corn syrup
		Milk chocolate

- **Beans and Legumes**

Consumption of beans and legumes is very important during the anti-inflammatory diet. They are rich in fiber and contain large amounts of protein as well as antioxidants. It is necessary to eat at least two servings of beans or legumes per week.

Note that beans and legumes can cause inflammation only if they are cooked in the wrong way. It is recommended to soak beans before cooking.

- **Others**

Fast food and processed food are forbidden during the anti-inflammatory diet. Such food damages our digestive and immune system.

Top 10 Anti-Inflammatory Diet Tips

- **Avoid white food**

Avoiding white food such as sugar, salt, etc. can help to maintain and control the normal level of blood sugar. Try to add more lean proteins and high fiber food to your daily diet. It can be lean types of meat, brown rice, and whole grains.

- **An apple a day keeps the doctors away**

Add vegetables, fruits, nuts, and spices to your daily meal plan. Garlic, ginger, cinnamon, and lemon will help to boost your immune system and reduce inflammation.

- **Exercise daily**

Regular sports activities can help to prevent inflammation. Do 5-10 minutes of exercise daily to feel healthier.

- **Balance your mind**

Everyday stress leads to chronic diseases. Practicing yoga, meditation, or biofeedback are excellent ways to balance your mind and manage stress.

- **Choose the right proteins**

Lean red meat can be served as a source of proteins but it is still high in cholesterol and salt. Instead, choose fish such as halibut, salmon, tuna, cod, or seabass. They are rich in omega-3 fatty acids.

- **Drink antioxidant beverages**

Herbs are a great source of antioxidants and promote faster treatment. Basil, thyme, oregano, chili pepper, and curcumin have high anti-inflammatory features and serve as natural painkillers.

- **Get enough sleep**

You should always get 8-9 hours of sleep at night. Too much or too little sleep is the main triggers for heart disease and type 2 diabetes.

- **Cross out alcohol from your diet**

Avoiding alcohol helps keep you calm and reduces the risk of inflammation.

Choose green tea instead of coffee or black tea.

Green tea can fight free radical damage. Drinking green tea regularly lowers the risk of cancer and Alzheimer's disease.

- **Consume probiotics every day**

Urban lifestyle and junk food is bad for your digestion. Eating food that is rich in probiotics like sauerkraut, yogurt, milk, kombucha, miso, kimchi, and fermented vegetables/fruits every day will improve your gut's microbe barrier.

BREAKFAST

Corn Bowl

4 Servings

Preparation Time: 10 minutes

Ingredients

- 10 oz corn Kernels, cooked
- 1 cup Tomatoes, chopped
- 1 tablespoon fresh dill, chopped
- 1 tablespoon plain Yogurt
- ½ cup Radish, chopped

Directions

- Mix Tomatoes with fresh dill, plain yogurt, and radish.
- Then add corn kernels, gently stir the meal.

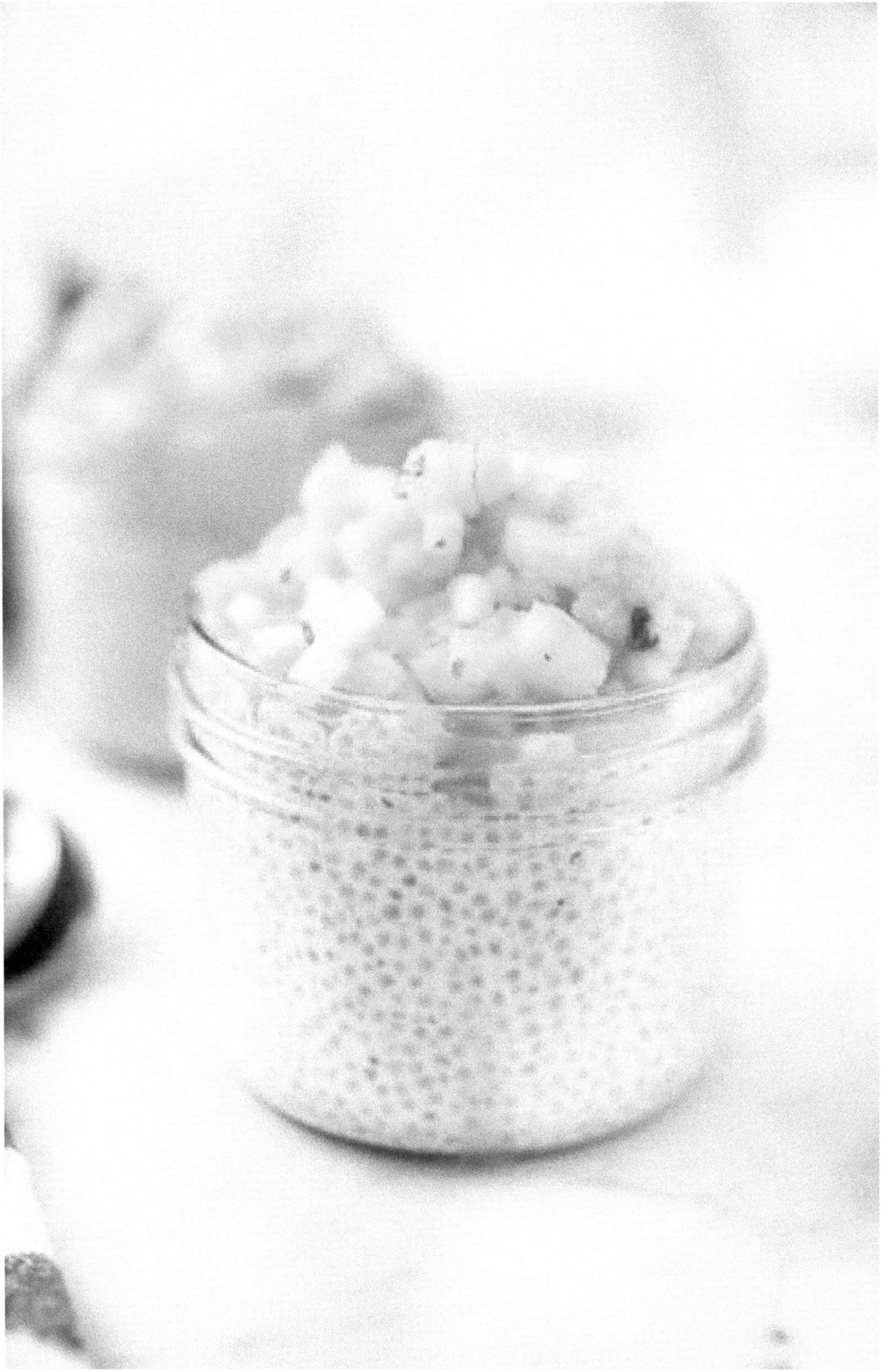

Lemon Tomatoes

6 Servings

Preparation Time: 10 minutes

Ingredients

- 4 cups Arugula , chopped
- 4 cups Tomatoes, chopped
- 2 tablespoons Olive oil
- 3 tablespoons Lemon juice
- 1 teaspoon Lemon zest, grated

Directions

- Add Tomatoes and Arugula in the mixing bowl.
- Add lemon juice, Olive oil, and lemon zest.
- Stir the meal gently before serving.

Blueberry Porridge

6 Servings

Preparation Time: 10minutes

Ingredients

- 4 tablespoons Chia seeds
- 1 cup Blueberries
- 3 cups Coconut cream
- 4 teaspoons raw Honey
- ½ teaspoon Vanilla extract

Directions

- Mix Coconut cream with chis seeds and raw honey.
- Blend the blueberries until smooth and add in the chia mixture.
- Then add vanilla extract, stir the porridge, and transfer in the serving bowls.

Nutmeg Oats

6 Servings

Preparation Time: 25 minutes

Ingredients

- 1 cup of Coconut milk
- ½ cup old-fashioned Oats
- 1 Pear, chopped
- 1 teaspoon ground Nutmeg
- 2 teaspoons raw Honey

Directions

- Bring the Coconut milk to boil and add Oats .
- Simmer them for 5 minutes.
- Then remove the Oats from the heat and add pear, ground nutmeg, and honey.
- Gently stir the meal.

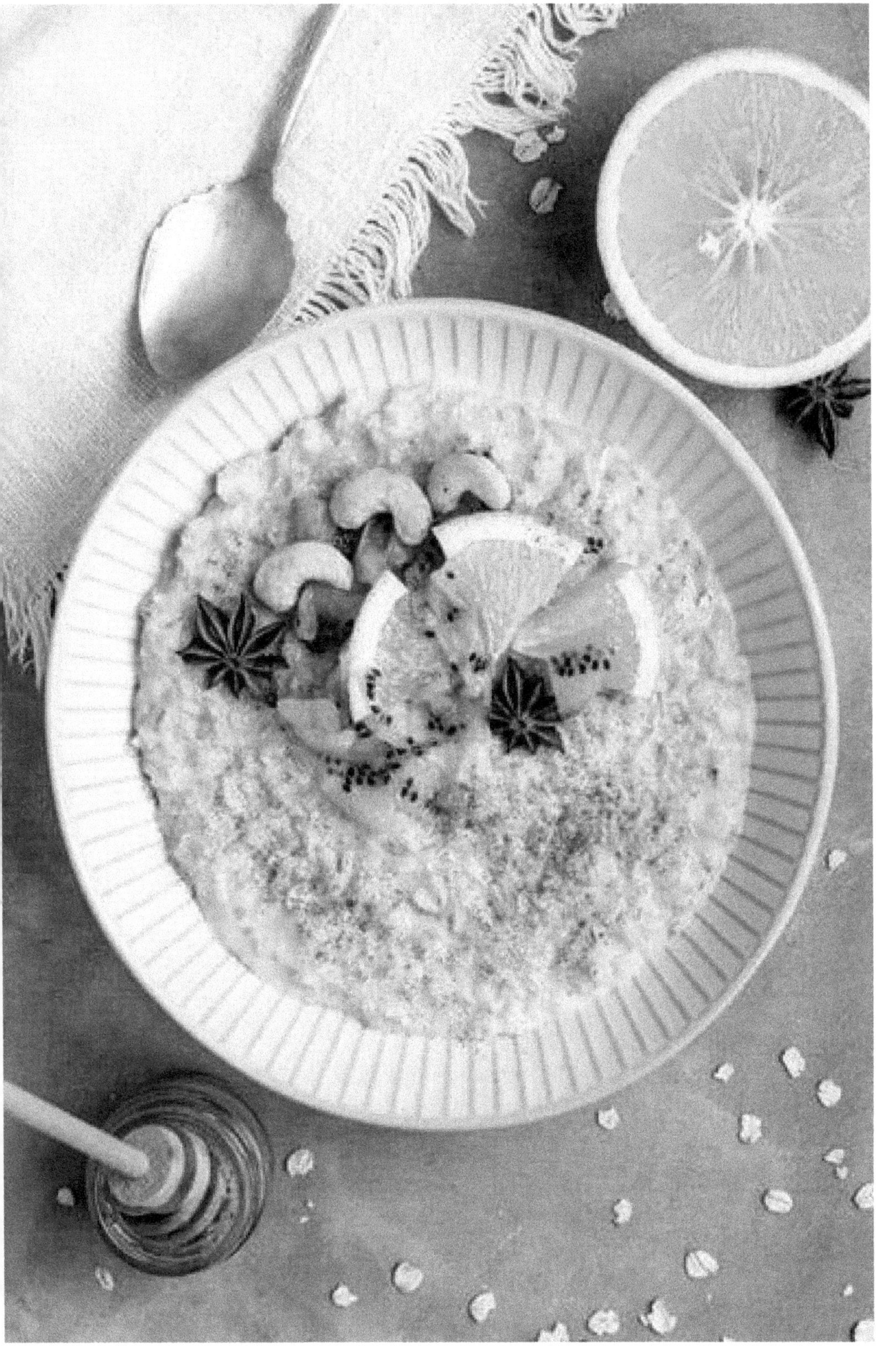

Pineapple Bowl

3 Servings

Preparation Time: 5minutes

Ingredients

- 1 cup Pineapple, peeled and cubed
- 1 Avocado, peeled, chopped
- 1 pear, cubed
- 1 teaspoon chia seeds
- 1 tablespoon lemon juice
- ½ tablespoon Avocado oil

Directions

- In the bowl, mix Pineapple with avocado, pear, lemon juice, and avocado oil.
- Shake the mixture and top with chia seeds.

Pumpkin Pie Spices Quinoa

5 Servings

Preparation Time: 10minutes

Ingredients

- 2 cups quinoa, cooked
- 1 tablespoon pumpkin pie spices
- 1 tablespoon raw honey

Directions

- Mix quinoa with pumpkin pie spices.
- Top the meal with raw honey.

Nutmeg Pork

6 Servings

Preparation Time: 55 minutes

Ingredients

- 1 tablespoon ground nutmeg
- 1 cup of Water
- 1-pound pork tenderloin, chopped
- 1 teaspoon dried rosemary

Directions

- Bring the Water to boil.
- Add ground nutmeg and dried rosemary.
- Then add pork tenderloin and close the lid.
- Simmer the meat on low heat for 35 minutes.

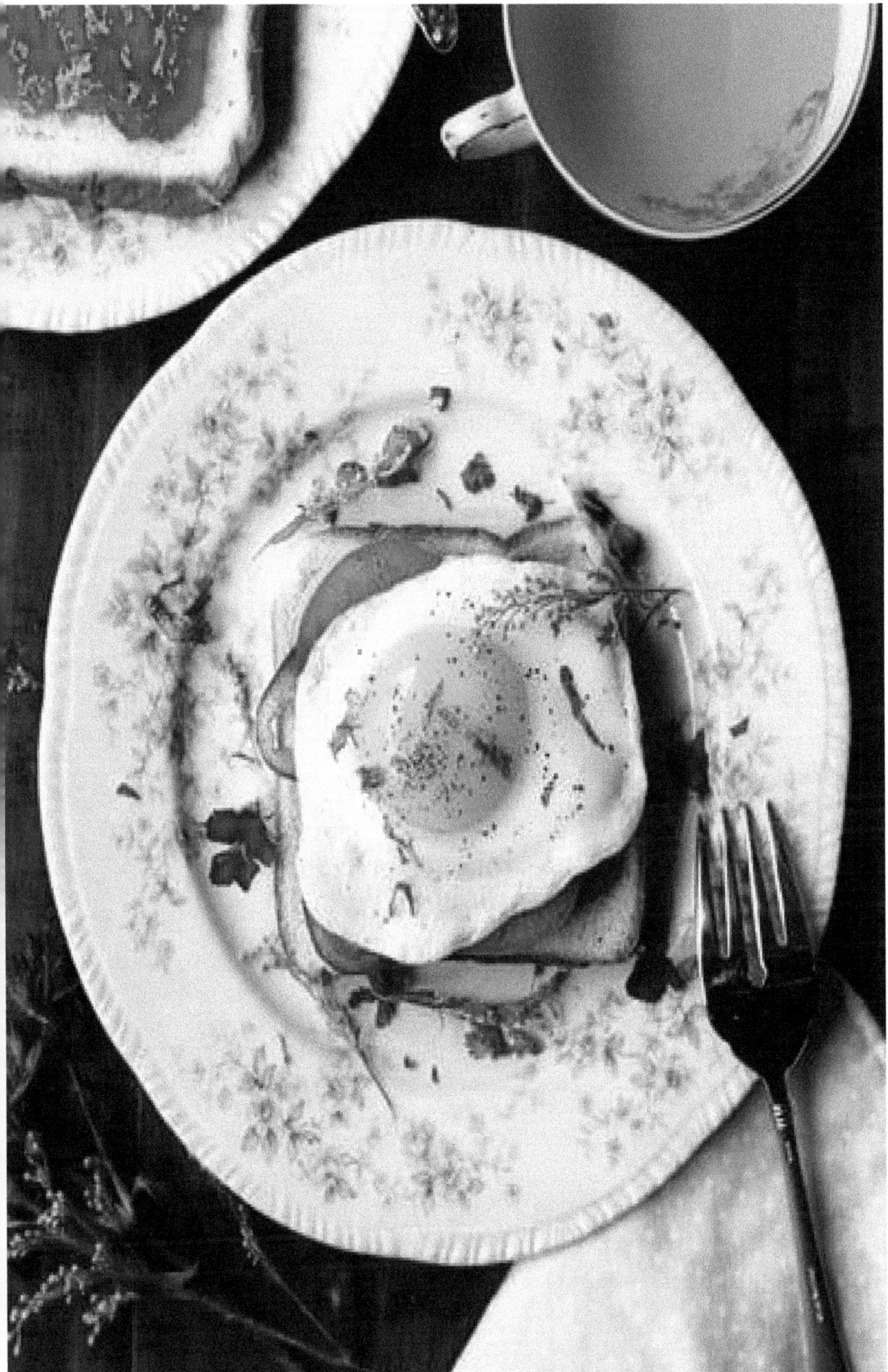

Rosemary Pork Cubes

6 Servings

Preparation Time: 50 minutes

Ingredients

- 2 pounds pork tenderloin, cubed
- 1 tablespoon dried rosemary
- 1 cup Tomatoes, chopped
- 4 Garlic cloves, chopped
- 2 cups of Water
- 1 tablespoon Olive oil

Directions

- In the mixing bowl, mix pork stew meat with dried rosemary, garlic, and Olive oil.
- Then add the mixture in the saucepan, add Tomatoes and Water.
- Close the lid and cook the meal on low heat for 40 minutes.

LUNCH

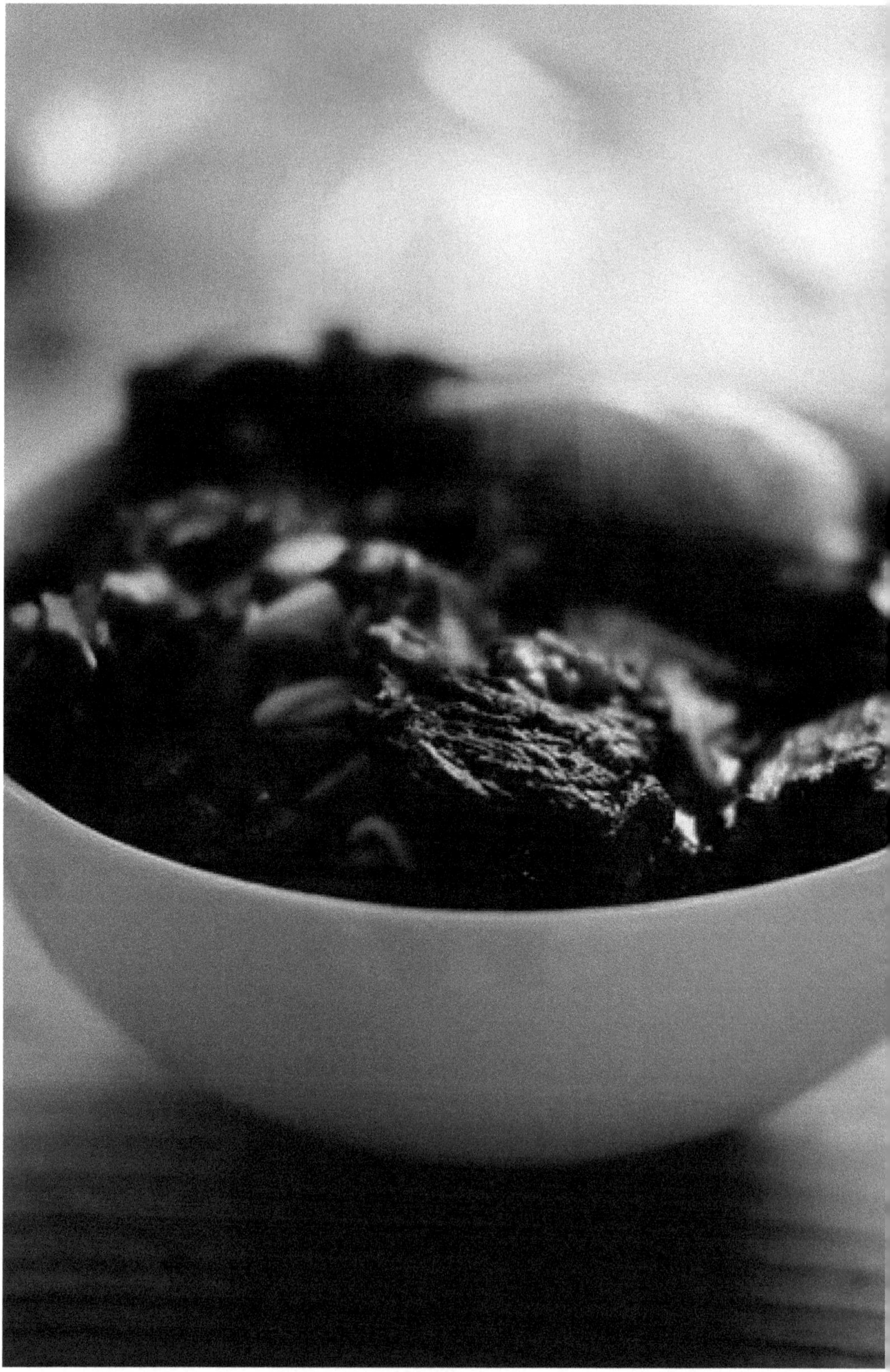

Cod and Tarragon Sauce

6 Servings

Preparation Time: 25 minutes

Ingredients

- 4 medium cod fillets, skinless and boneless
- 2 tablespoons mustard
- 1 tablespoon chopped tarragon
- 1 tablespoon capers, drained
- 4 tablespoons Olive oil+ 1 teaspoon
- Salt and black pepper to the taste
- 2 cups lettuce leaves, torn
- 1 small red onion, sliced
- 1 small cucumber, sliced
- 2 tablespoons lemon juice
- 2 tablespoons Water

Directions

- In a bowl, mix mustard with 2 tablespoons Olive oil, tarragon, capers and Water, whisk well and set aside.
- Heat up a pan with 1 teaspoon oil over medium-high heat.
- Season fish with salt and pepper to the taste, then add to pan and cook for 6 minutes on each side. In a separate bowl, mix cucumber with onion, lettuce, lemon juice, 2 tablespoons Olive oil, salt and pepper to the taste. Arrange the cod between plates drizzle the tarragon sauce all over, and serve with the cucumber salad on the side.

Orange Chicken Salad

3 Servings

Preparation Time: 40 minutes

Ingredients

- 1 whole chicken, cut into medium pieces
- 4 scallions, chopped
- 2 celery ribs, chopped
- 1 cup chopped mandarin orange
- ¼ cup avocado mayonnaise
- ½ cup Coconut cream
- 1 cup chopped cashews, toasted
- A pinch of salt and black pepper

Directions

- Add Chicken pieces in a pot and add Water to cover.
- Add a pinch of salt then bring to a boil over medium heat and cook for 25 minutes.

- Transfer to a cutting board, discard bones, shred meat and Add in a bowl.
- Add celery, orange pieces, cashews, scallion, salt, pepper, mayo and the Coconut cream, toss to coat and serve.

Brown Rice with Chicken

6 Servings

Preparation Time: 20 minutes

Ingredients

- 1½ cups brown rice, cooked
- 1½ tablespoons Coconut sugar
- 1 cup Chicken stock
- 2 tablespoon Coconut aminos
- 4 ounces Chicken breast boneless, skinless and cut into small pieces
- 1 egg
- 2 egg whites
- 2 scallions, chopped

Directions

- Add stock in a pot, heat up over medium-low heat and add Coconut aminos and sugar, stir, bring to a boil, add the Chicken and toss.

- In a bowl, mix the egg with egg whites, whisk well then add over the Chicken mix.
- Sprinkle the scallions on top and cook for 3 minutes without stirring.
- Divide the rice into 4 bowls, add the Chicken mix on top and serve.

Greek Chicken Breasts

6 Servings

Preparation Time: 40 minutes

Ingredients

- 6 Chicken breast halves, skinless and boneless
- 2 teaspoons Olive oil
- ½ cup vegetable stock
- 1 tablespoon chopped basil
- 2 teaspoons chopped thyme
- ½ cup chopped yellow Onion
- 3 Garlic cloves, minced
- ½ cup kalamata olives, pitted and sliced
- ¼ cup chopped Parsley
- 3 cups chopped Tomatoes

Directions

- Heat up a pan with the oil over medium heat, add Chicken and cook for 6 minutes on each side.

- Transfer cooked Chicken to a plate. Heat up the same pan used for the Chicken over medium heat, add garlic, stir and cook for 1 minute.
- Add onion, Tomatoes, and the stock, then stir and bring to a simmer. Cook for 10 minutes.
- Add basil, thyme and the chicken, mix and cook for 12 minutes. Add parsley, olives, salt and pepper, toss, divide between plates and serve.

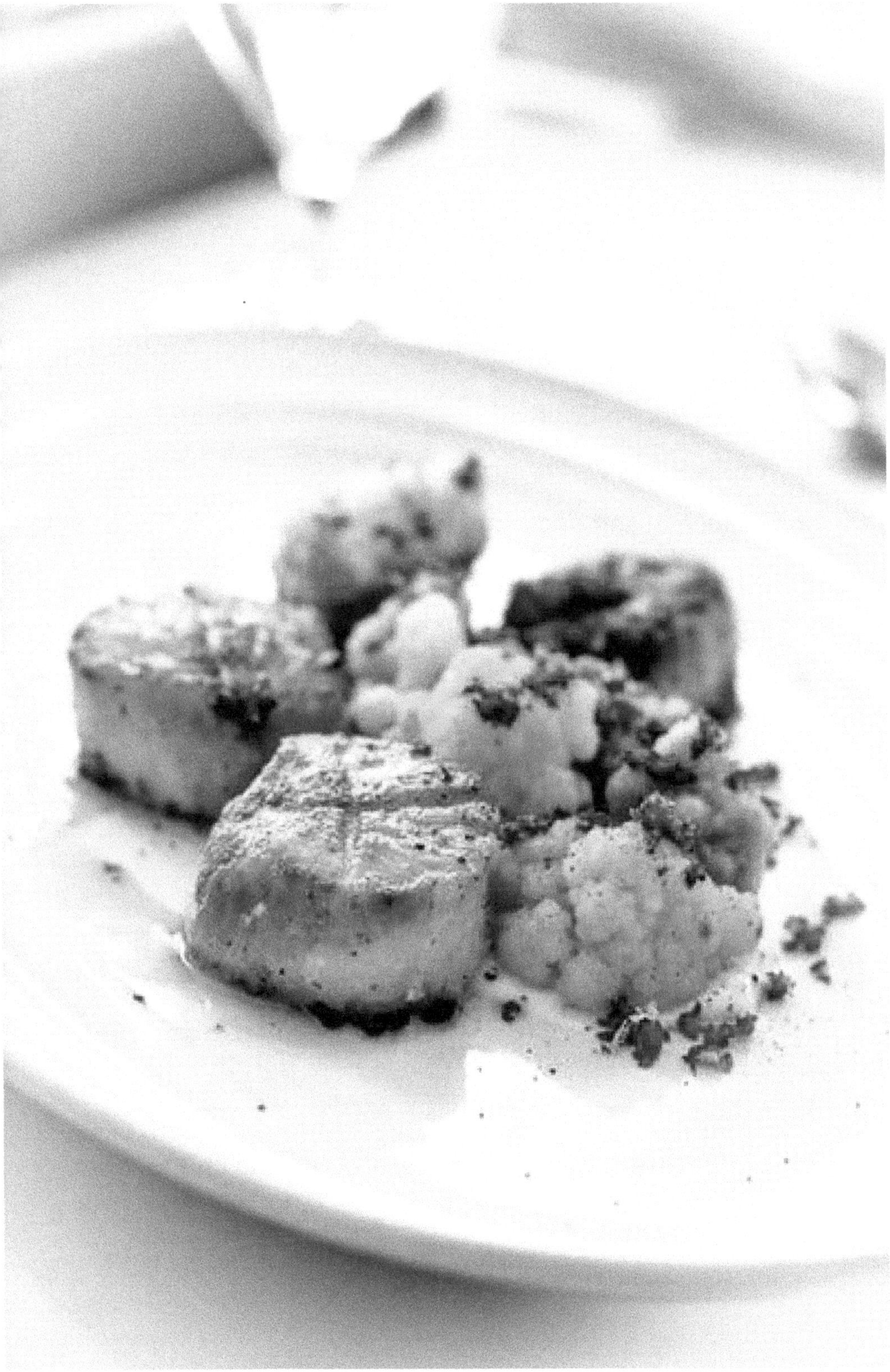

Easy Chicken with Potato

5 Servings

Preparation Time: 1 hour

Ingredients

- 1 tablespoon Olive oil
- 4 teaspoons garlic, minced
- A pinch of salt and black pepper
- ¼ teaspoon dried thyme
- 12 small red potatoes, halved
- Cooking spray
- 2 pounds Chicken breast, skinless, boneless and cubed
- 1 cup sliced red Onion
- ¾ cup vegetable stock
- ½ cup pepperoncini peppers, chopped
- 2 cups chopped tomato
- ¼ cup kalamata olives, pitted and halved
- 2 tablespoons chopped basil
- 14 ounces canned artichokes, drained and chopped

Directions

- In a baking dish, mix potatoes with 2 teaspoons garlic, Olive oil, thyme, salt and pepper.
- Bake in the oven at 400 degrees ° for 30 minutes.
- Heat up a pot over medium-high heat, grease with cooking spray, add chicken, season with salt and black pepper and cook for 5 minutes on each side, then transfer to a plate.
- Heat up the pot again over medium heat, add onion, stir and cook for 5 minutes
- Add stock and return the Chicken to the pot. Add olives, pepperoncini and roasted potatoes, stir and cook for 3 minutes. Add the rest of the garlic, artichokes, basil and the Tomatoes, stir, cook for 3 minutes. Divide between plates and serve.

Paprika Chicken Mix

6 Servings

Preparation Time: 40 minutes

Ingredients

- 1/3 cup mustard
- Salt and black pepper to the taste
- 1 cup yellow onion, chopped
- 1 tablespoon Olive oil
- 1 and ½ cups Chicken stock
- 4 Chicken breasts, skinless and boneless
- ¼ teaspoon sweet paprika

Directions

- In a bowl, whisk the paprika with mustard, salt and pepper.
- Spread the mix over the Chicken and rub well.
- Heat up a pan with the oil over medium-high heat, add Chicken breasts and cook for 2 minutes on each side, then transfer to a plate.

- Heat up the pan once again over medium-high heat, add stock, stir and bring to a simmer.
- Add onions, salt, pepper and return the Chicken to the pan as well. Stir the mix and bring to a simmer over medium heat for 20 minutes, turning meat halfway.
- Divide between plates, drizzle the sauce over it and serve.

Grilled Eggplant Salad

6 Servings

Preparation Time: 30 minutes

Ingredients

- 1 tomato, diced
- 1 eggplant, pricked
- A pinch of salt and black pepper
- ¼ teaspoon ground turmeric
- 1½ teaspoons red wine vinegar
- ½ teaspoon chopped oregano
- 3 tablespoons Olive oil
- 2 Garlic cloves, minced
- 3 tablespoons chopped Parsley
- 2 tablespoons chopped capers

Directions

- Heat up your grill over medium-high heat, add eggplant, cook for 15 minutes, turning from time to time, scoop flesh, roughly chop and Add in a bowl.
- Add salt, pepper to the taste, Tomatoes, turmeric, garlic, vinegar, oregano, parsley, oil and capers, toss and serve.

Eggplant with Avocado Lunch

6 Servings

Preparation Time: 20 minutes

Ingredients

- 1 eggplant, sliced
- 1 red onion, sliced
- 2 teaspoons Olive oil
- 1 Avocado, pitted and chopped
- 1 teaspoon mustard
- 1 tablespoon red wine vinegar
- 1 tablespoon chopped oregano
- 1 teaspoon raw honey
- A pinch of salt and black pepper
- 1 tablespoon chopped Parsley
- Zest of 1 lemon

Directions

- Brush the Onion slices and eggplant slices with the Olive oil, place them on the preheated kitchen grill, cook for 5 minutes on each side and let cool down.
- Cut the veggies into cubes; add in a mixing bowl, add avocado and toss. In a bowl, mix vinegar with mustard, oregano, honey, Olive oil, salt and pepper, whisk well and add to the salad.
- Toss together and sprinkle the lemon zest and the Parsley on top and serve.

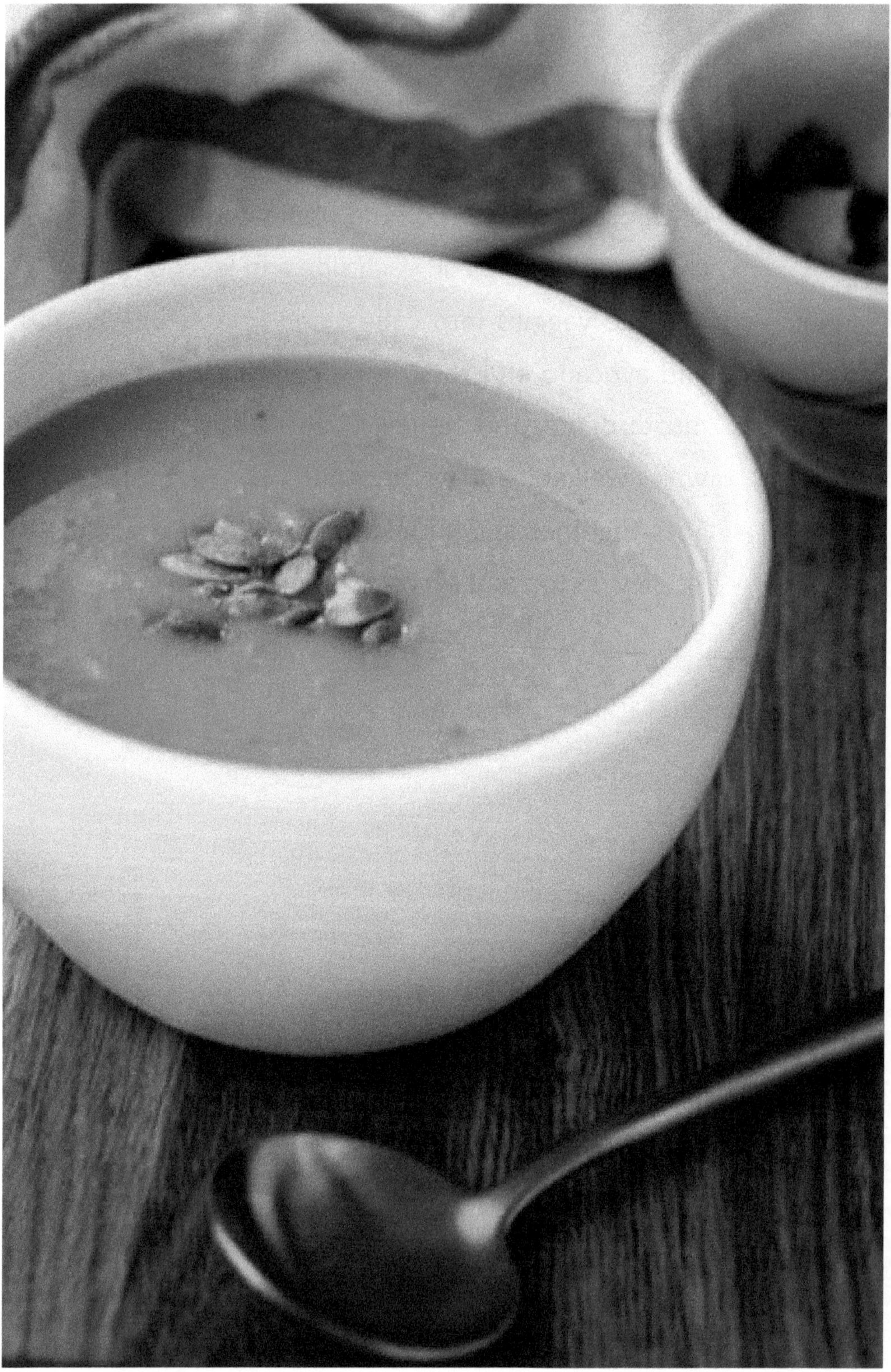

Eggplant with Egg

6 Servings

Preparation Time: 40 minutes

Ingredients

- 1 big purple eggplant, cubed
- ¼ cup Olive oil
- 12 eggs, hard-boiled, peeled and cubed
- Juice of 1 lemon
- A pinch of salt and white pepper
- 1/3 cup pine nuts
- ¼ cup mustard
- 1 cup chopped sun-dried Tomatoes
- 1 cup halved walnuts

Directions

- Spread eggplant cubes on a lined baking sheet. In a bowl, whisk together half of the lemon juice with the oil, salt and pepper.

- Pour the mix over the eggplant cubes, toss to coat, introduce in the oven at 400 degrees ° and bake for 30 minutes.
- In a food processor, mix the rest of the lemon juice, mustard, salt, pepper, walnuts, Tomatoes and pine nuts and pulse well.
- Add the eggs in a bowl, add eggplant cubes, mustard mix, toss to coat well and serve.

SNACKS & APPETIZERS

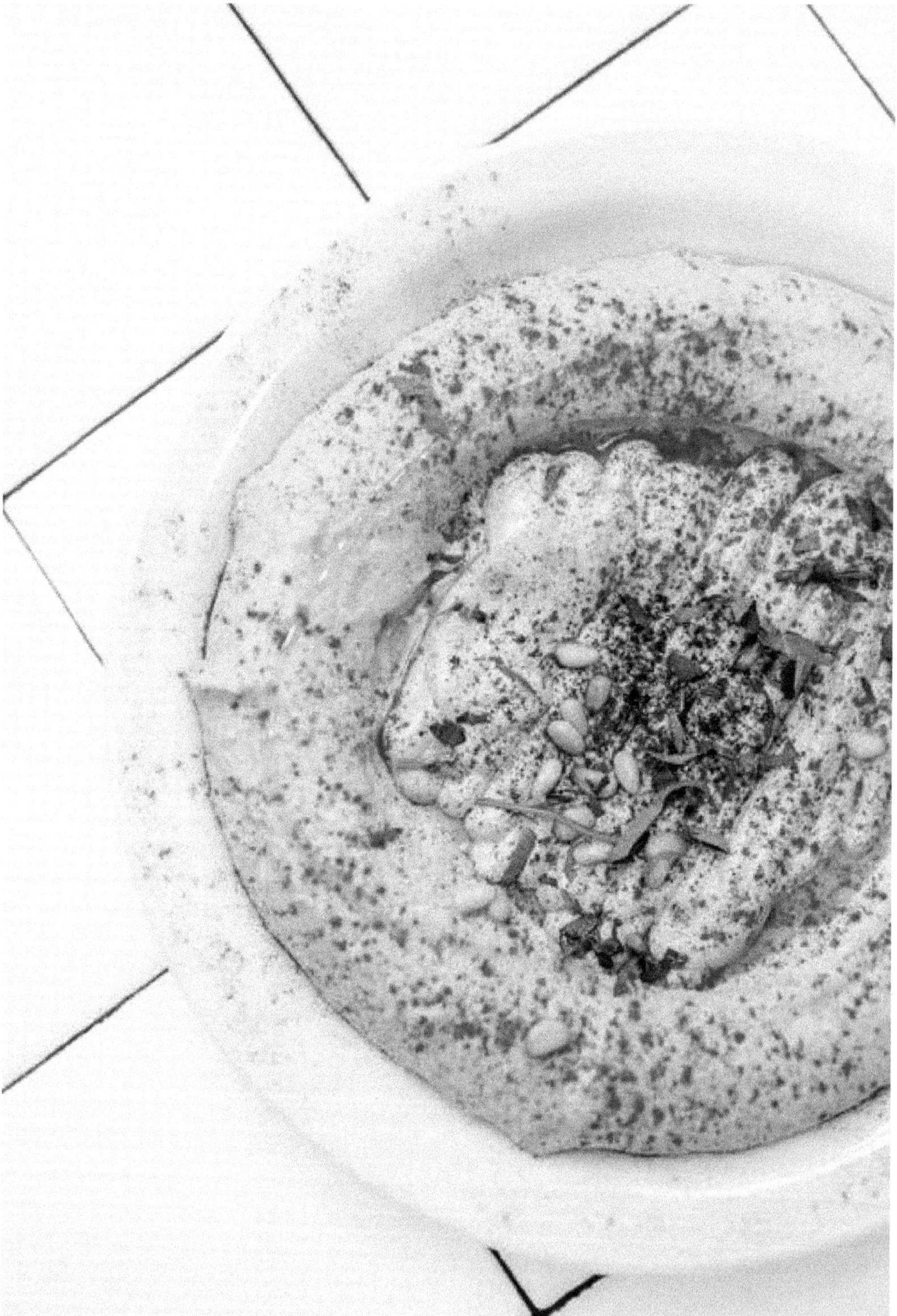

Simple Peanut Butter Dip

6 Servings

Preparation time: 10 minutes

Ingredients

- ½ cup Coconut cream
- ¼ cup Peanut butter, soft

Directions

- In a bowl, mix together the peanut butter with the coconut cream.
- Divide into bowls and serve.

Easy Nutmeg Apple Snack

6 Servings

Preparation time: 2hours 10minutes

Ingredients

- 2 Apples, cored and cubed
- A pinch of ground Nutmeg
- Cooking spray
- Ground Cinnamon to taste

Directions

- Arrange the apple cubes on a lined baking sheet and sprinkle with cinnamon, nutmeg and spray with the cooking oil.
- Toss the apples slices well and place in the oven at 275°F. Bake for 2 hours.
- Divide into bowls and serve as a snack

Dill Coconut Dip

6 Servings

Preparation time: 10minutes

Ingredients

- 1 teaspoon Sweet paprika
- 2 teaspoons sun-dried Tomatoes, chopped
- 2 teaspoons dried Parsley
- 2 teaspoons chopped Chives
- A pinch of sea Salt and Black pepper
- 1½ cups Coconut cream
- 2 teaspoons dried Dill
- 2 teaspoons dried Thyme

Directions

- In a bowl, mix the coconut cream with the dill, thyme, paprika, tomatoes, parsley, chives, salt and pepper and serve cold as a snack.

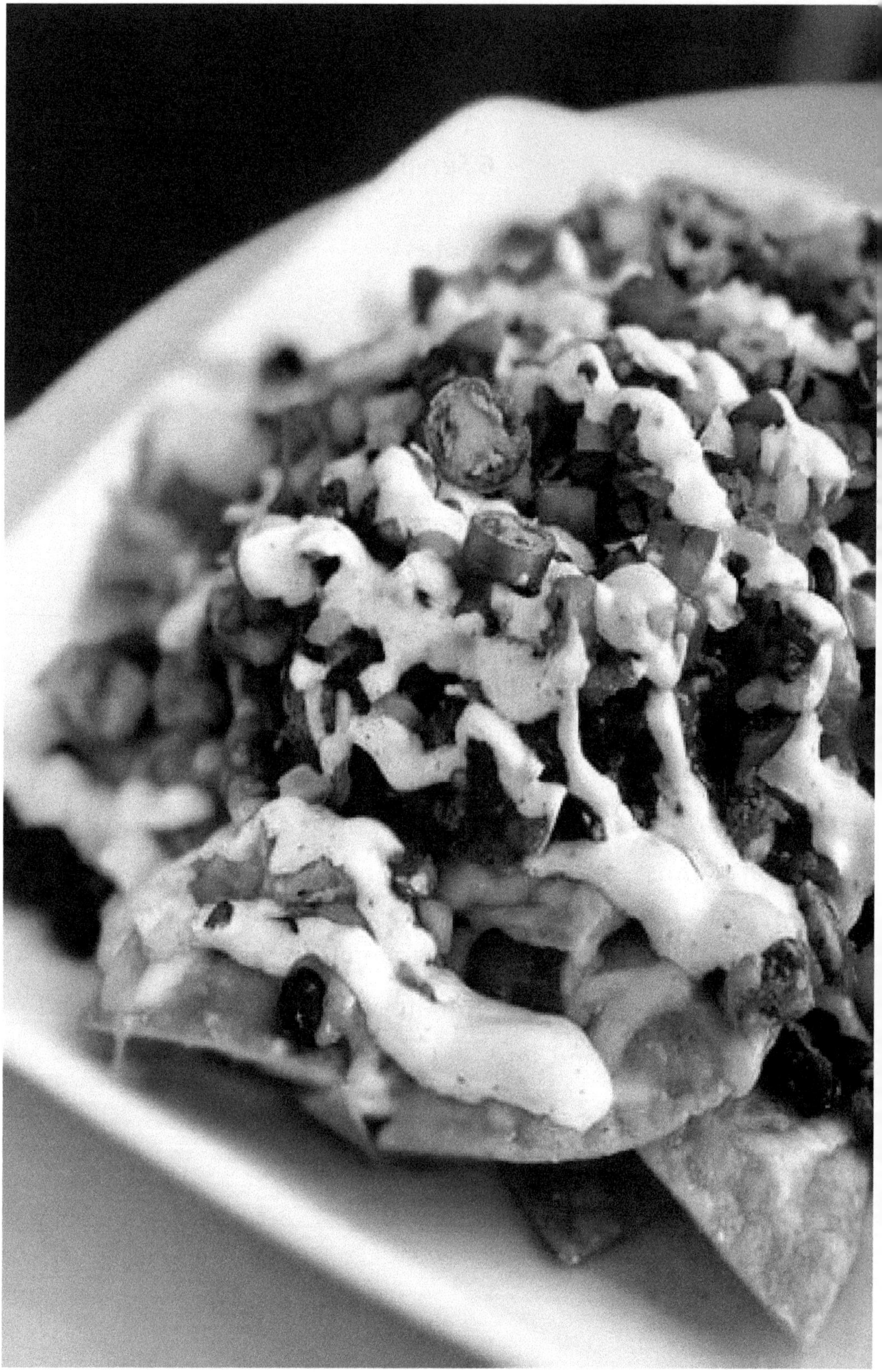

Sweet Potato and Sesame Spread

6 Servings

Preparation time: 25minutes

Ingredients

- 1 tablespoon Olive oil
- 5 Garlic cloves, minced
- ½ teaspoon Ground cumin
- 2 tablespoons Water
- A pinch of Salt
- 1 cup canned Garbanzo beans, drained and rinsed
- 4 cups chopped, peeled Sweet potatoes
- ¼ cup Sesame paste
- 2 tablespoons Lime juice

Directions

- Put the sweet potatoes in a steamer basket, add some water into a pot and place the basket on top.
- Bring to a boil over medium-high heat and steam potatoes for 15 minutes.

- Drain, let them cool and then put them into a blender. Add the sesame paste, garlic, beans, lemon juice, cumin, water, salt and oil.
- Blend it well, transfer to bowls and serve.

Dill Zucchini Patties

8 Servings

Preparation time: 30minutes

Ingredients

- 2 Garlic cloves, minced
- 3 Zucchinis, grated and excess water squeezed
- Cooking spray
- ½ cup chopped Dill
- 1 Egg
- ½ cup Coconut flour
- A pinch of sea Salt and Black pepper
- 1 yellow Onion, chopped

Directions

- In a bowl, mix the zucchinis with garlic, onion, flour, salt, pepper, egg and dill.
- Shape medium patties out of this mix and arrange them on a lined baking sheet.

- Spray them with cooking oil, and bake in the oven at 400°F for 10 minutes on each side.
- Arrange the patties on a platter and serve as an appetizer.

Simple Cauliflower Crackers

8 Servings

Preparation time: 50 minutes

Ingredients

- 1 teaspoon Italian seasoning
- A pinch of sea Salt and Black pepper
- Black pepper to the taste
- 1 big Cauliflower head, florets separated
- ¼ cup Egg whites

Directions

- Put the cauliflower florets in a blender and blend until you obtain your cauliflower "rice" then spread the rice on a lined baking sheet.
- Place in the oven at 375 °F, roast for 20 minutes, then put in a clean bowl, squeezing to remove any excess moisture.
- Mix in salt, pepper, Italian seasoning and egg whites.

- Spread this into a lined rectangular pan and press well. Place in the oven at 375° F and bake for 20 minutes.
- Cut into medium crackers and serve them cold.

Baked Mushroom Caps

4 Servings

Preparation time: 25minutes

Ingredients

- Black pepper to the taste
- 2-pound brown Mushrooms, stems discarded
- A pinch of sea Salt and Black pepper

Directions

- Arrange the mushroom caps on a lined baking sheet, season them with a pinch of salt and black pepper and place in the oven at 400 degrees F.
- Bake for 15 minutes and divide into bowls to serve cold.

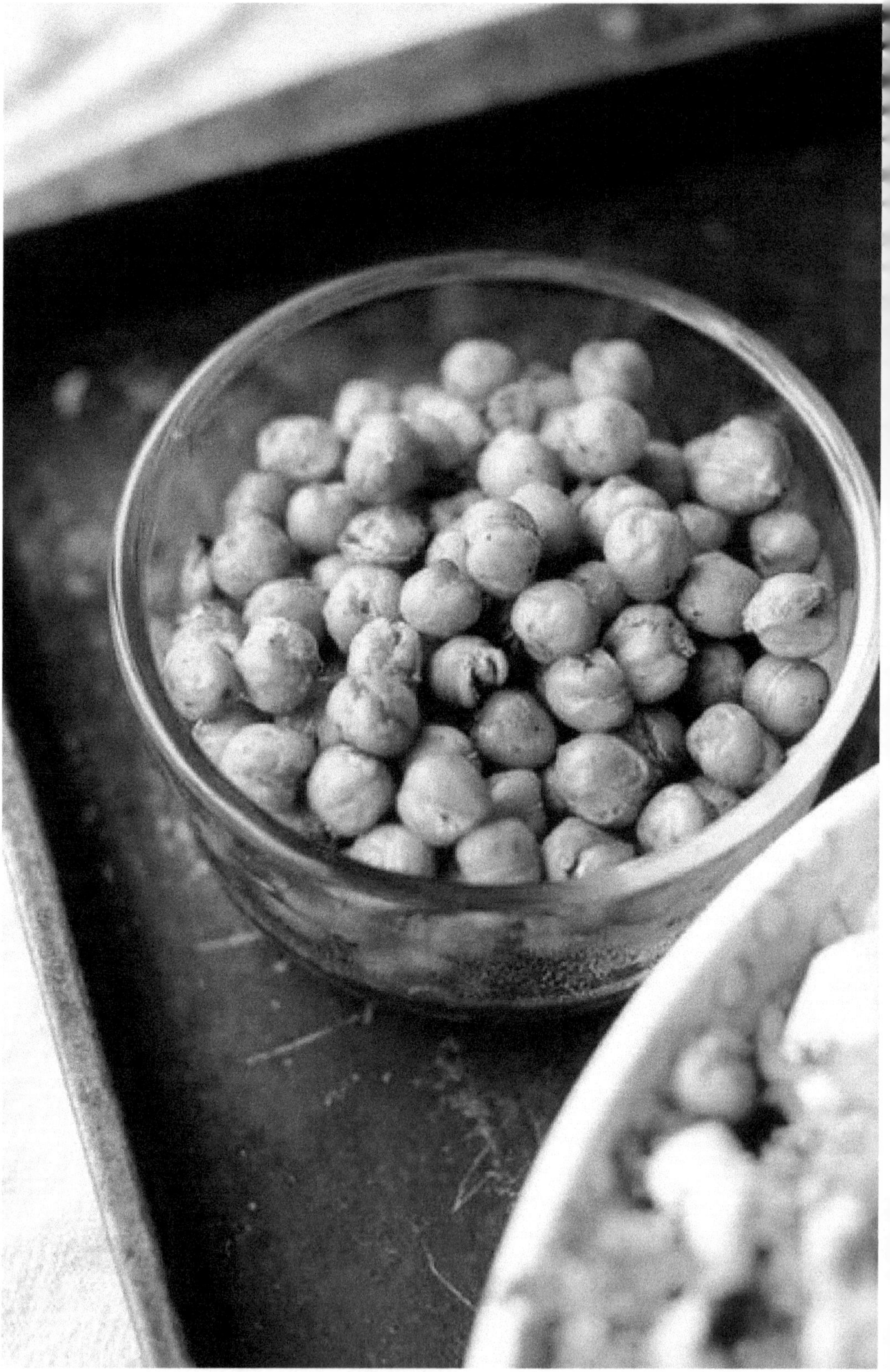

Almond Spinach Dip

8 Servings

Preparation time: 45 minutes

Ingredients

- 4 Garlic cloves, minced
- ½ cup chopped Green onions
- A pinch of Black pepper
- 1 tablespoon Oregano, dried
- Cooking spray
- ½ cup Almond milk
- 1½ cups Coconut cream
- 10 ounces Spinach

Directions

- In a bowl, mix the spinach with the almond milk, cream, garlic, green onions, oregano and black pepper.

- Spray a baking dish with cooking oil and spread the spinach dip in the pan, introduce in the oven at 350 degrees F and bake for 35 minutes.
- Leave your dip to cool down a bit before serving it.

DINNER

Baked Leek

6 Servings

Preparation Time: 30 minutes

Ingredients

- 1-pound leek, sliced
- 1 carrot, grated
- 1 cup of Coconut milk
- 1 teaspoon Olive oil
- 1 teaspoon ground black pepper

Directions

- Mix leek with grated carrot, Olive oil, ground black pepper, and Coconut milk.
- Add the mixture in the baking pan and flatten it gently.
- Bake the meal at 365° for 20 minutes.

Broccoli Steaks

4 Servings

Preparation Time: 30 minutes

Ingredients

- 1-pound Broccoli head
- 1 teaspoon Cayenne pepper
- 2 tablespoons Olive oil

Directions

- Slice the broccoli head into the steaks and Add in the baking tray in one layer.
- Sprinkle the vegetables with cayenne pepper and Olive oil.
- Bake the broccoli steaks at 365° for 10 minutes per side.

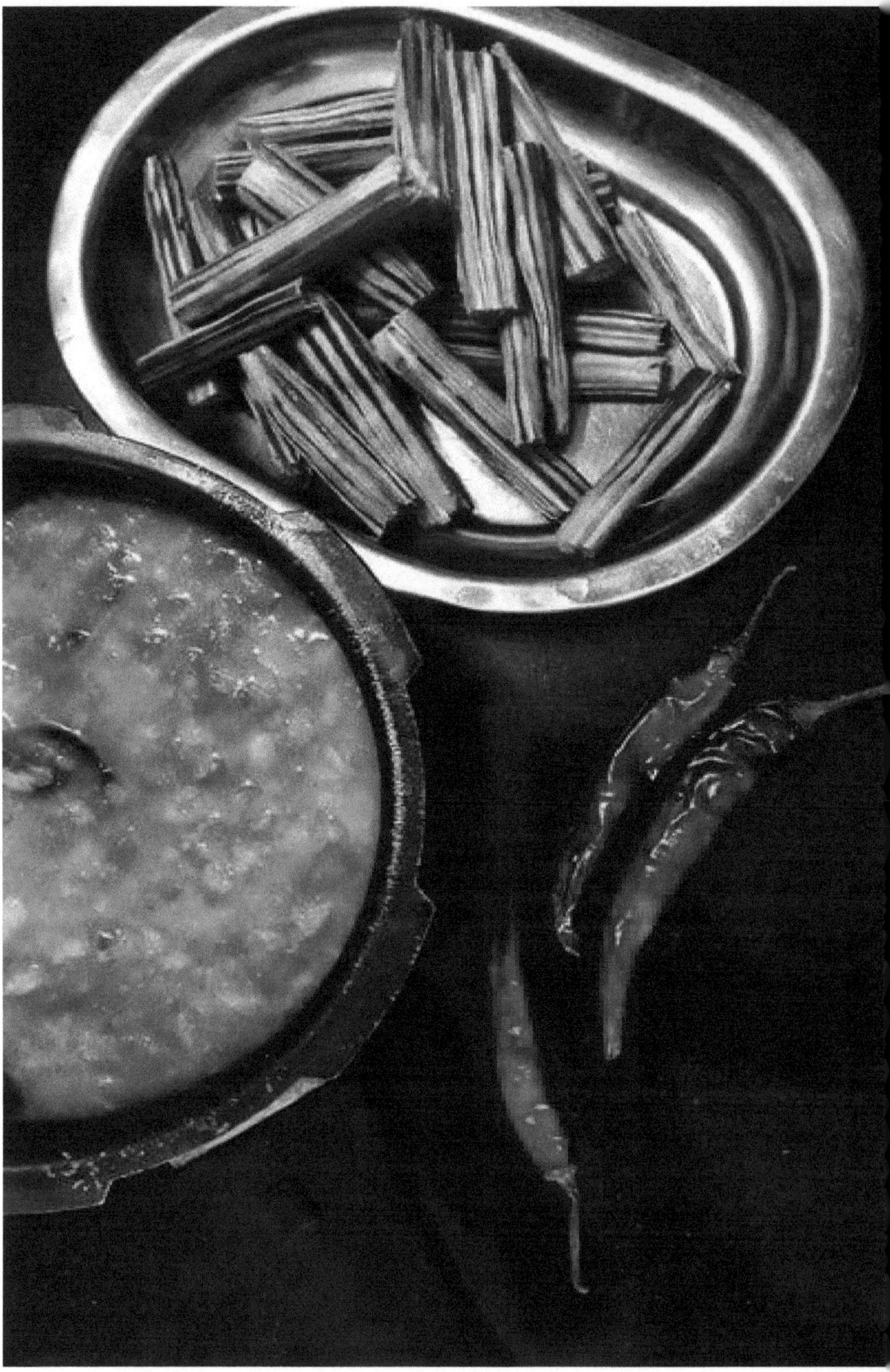

Thyme Haddock

6 Servings

Preparation Time: 20 minutes

Ingredients

- 1-pound Haddock fillets
- 1 tablespoon dried Thyme
- 1 tablespoon Olive oil
- 1 teaspoon Lemon zest, grated

Directions

- Mix fish with dried thyme, Olive oil, and lemon zest.
- Add the fish in the preheated to 400° grill and cook it for 4 minutes per side.

Nutmeg Trout

3 Servings

Preparation Time: 20 minutes

Ingredients

- 12 oz Trout fillet
- 2 tablespoons Olive oil
- 1 tablespoon Lemon juice
- 1 teaspoon Ground Nutmeg

Directions

- Rub the trout fillet with lemon juice and ground nutmeg.
- Then brush it with Olive oil and add it in the hot pan.
- Roast the fish for 5 minutes per side.

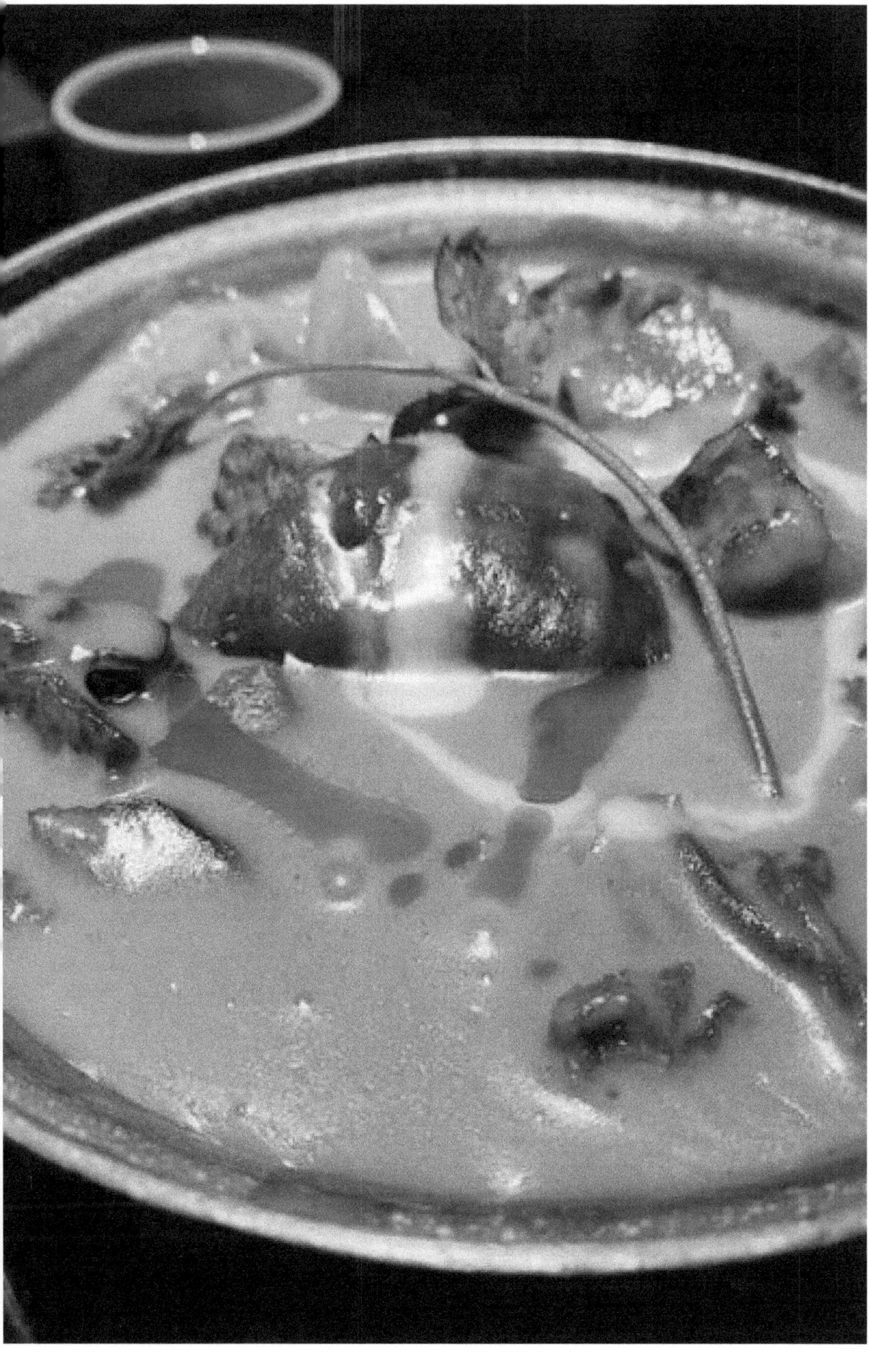

Cayenne Pepper Shrimps

6 Servings

Preparation Time: 20 minutes

Ingredients

- 2-pound Shrimps, peeled
- 1 tablespoon Olive oil
- 1 tablespoon Cayenne pepper
- 2 tablespoons Lemon juice

Directions

- Mix shrimps with Olive oil, lemon juice, and cayenne pepper.
- Preheat the pan well and add the shrimps inside.
- Cook them for 3 minutes per side.

Tomato Calamari

6 Servings

Preparation Time: 25 minutes

Ingredients

- 2-pounds Calamari, sliced
- 2 tablespoons Olive oil
- 1 cup Tomatoes
- 1 Chili pepper, chopped

Directions

- Mix Olive oil with chopped Tomatoes and add them in the saucepan.
- Roast the mixture for 5 minutes.
- Add chili pepper and calamari. Carefully mix the ingredients.
- Close the lid and cook the seafood for 10 minutes.

Chicken and Beans

6 Servings

Preparation Time: 45 minutes

Ingredients

- 1 cup red kidney beans, cooked
- 1-pound Chicken fillet, chopped
- 1 cup of Water
- 1 cup Tomatoes, chopped
- 1 teaspoon chili powder

Directions

- Add the Chicken fillet in the saucepan.
- Add red kidney beans, Water, Tomatoes, and chili powder.
- Close the lid and cook the meal on medium heat for 30 minutes.

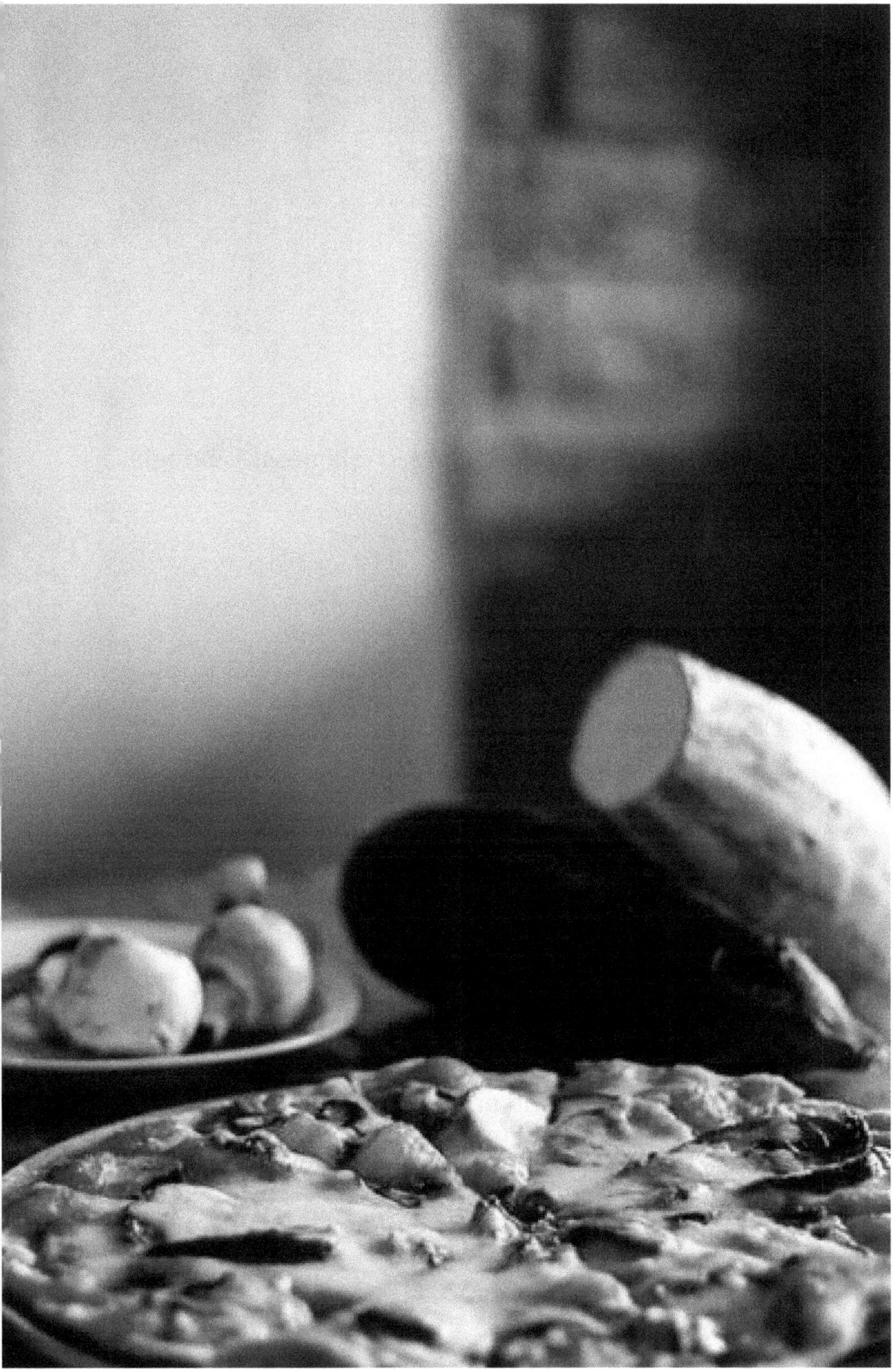

Chicken with Green Beans

6 Servings

Preparation Time: 50 minutes

Ingredients

- 12 oz green beans, chopped
- 1-pound Chicken thighs, skinless, boneless, chopped
- 1 teaspoon chili powder
- 2 tablespoons lemon juice
- 2 tablespoons Olive oil
- ¼ cup of Water

Directions

- Mix Chicken thighs with chili powder, lemon juice, and Olive oil.
- Preheat the saucepan and Add the Chicken inside. Roast it for 5 minutes per side.
- Then add Water and green beans.
- Close the lid and cook the meal on medium heat for 30 minutes.

Chicken and Beets

6 Servings

Preparation Time: 50 minutes

Ingredients

- 10 oz beets, peeled, chopped
- 1-pound Chicken breast, skinless, boneless, chopped
- 1 cup of Water
- 1 teaspoon dried rosemary
- 1 tablespoon Olive oil
- 1 teaspoon ground clove

Directions

- Roast the Chicken breast with oil for 5 minutes per side.
- Then Add the Chicken in the saucepan.
- Add beets, Water, dried rosemary, and ground clove.
- Close the lid and cook the meal for 30 minutes.

SOUPS

Sweet Soup

5 Servings

Preparation Time: 50 minutes

Ingredients

- 1 cup pumpkin, chopped.
- 3 cups tomatoes, chopped.
- 1 cup of water
- 1 teaspoon ground nutmeg
- 1 teaspoon olive oil

Directions

- Mix pumpkin with olive oil and roast for 2-3 minutes per side.
- Then put the pumpkin in the saucepan.
- Add tomatoes, water, and ground nutmeg.
- Cook the soup for 20 minutes on medium heat.
- Then blend it until smooth with the help of the immersion blender.
- Ladle the cooked soup in the bowls.

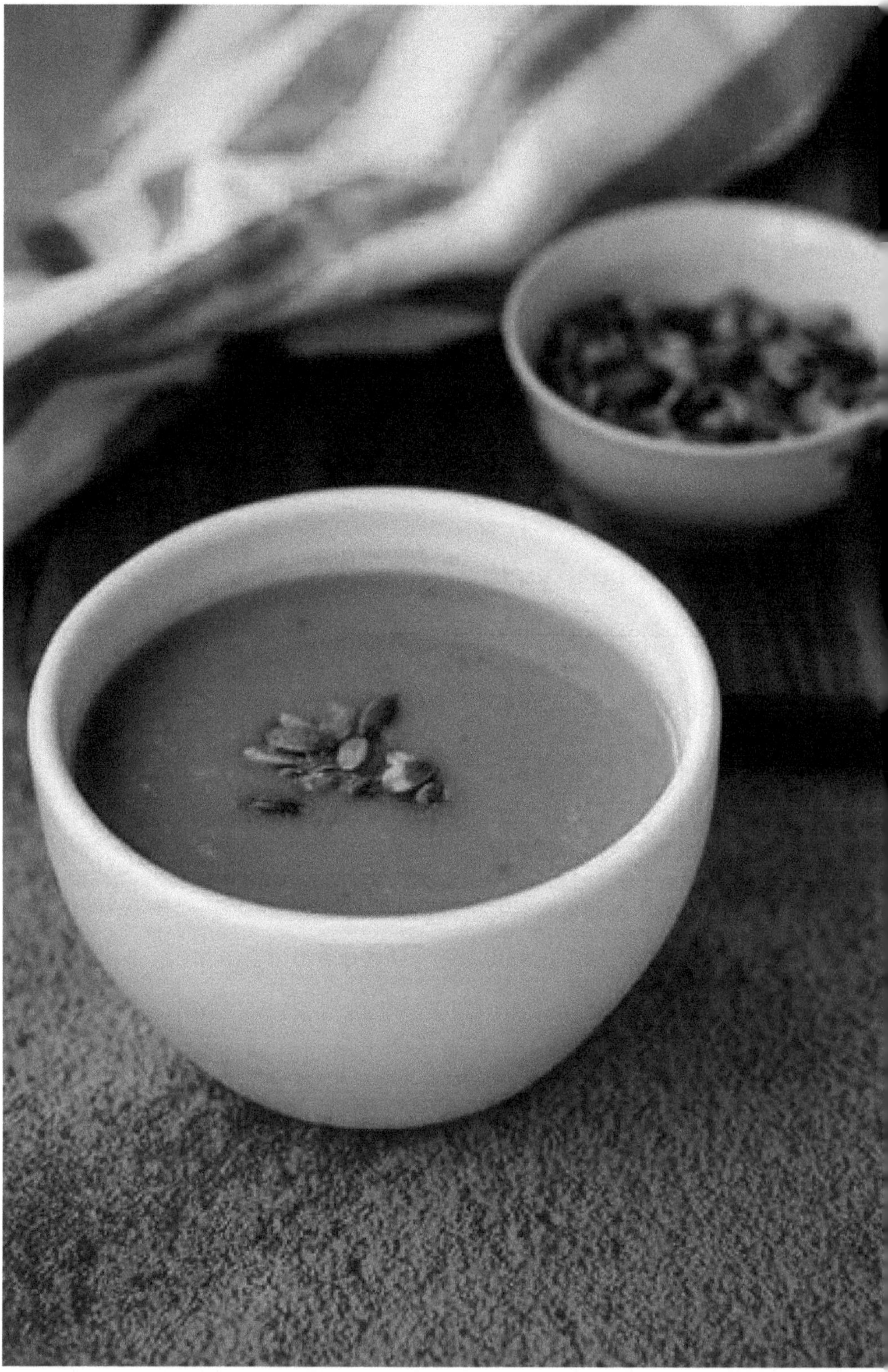

Parsnip Cream Soup

6 Servings

Preparation Time: 55 minutes

Ingredients

- 3 cups parsnip, chopped.
- 1 cup cauliflower, chopped.
- 1 teaspoon minced. garlic
- 1 teaspoon dried dill
- 4 cups of water
- 1 teaspoon ground clove
- 1 tablespoon olive oil

Directions

- Mix cauliflower with olive oil and roast it for 2 minutes per side.
- Then put the cauliflower in the saucepan. Add parsnip, minced. Garlic and dried dill.
- Add water and ground clove.
- Cook the soup for 30 minutes on low heat.

- When all ingredients of the soup are soft, blend the soup with the help of immersion blender.
- When the soup is smooth, it is cooked.

Wedges Soup

6 Servings

Preparation Time: 45 minutes

Ingredients

- 1 sweet pepper
- 1 zucchini
- 1 eggplant
- 1 tablespoon olive oil
- 1 teaspoon cayenne pepper
- 2 tbsps plain yogurt
- 4 cups of water

Directions

- Cut eggplant, zucchini, and sweet pepper into the wedges.
- Then put all vegetables in the saucepan and sprinkle with olive oil.
- Roast the vegetables for 5 minutes.

- Then mix them well and add cayenne pepper, plain yogurt, and water. Mix the mixture.
- Close the lid and cook the soup for 10 minutes on medium heat.

Curry Soup

6 Servings

Preparation Time: 35 minutes

Ingredients

- 1 tablespoon curry paste
- 4 cups of water
- 1 cup of coconut milk
- 1-pound cod, chopped.
- 1 cup onion, chopped.
- 1 tablespoon olive oil

Directions

- Mix curries paste with coconut milk.
- Then pour olive oil in the saucepan.
- Add onion and roast it for 2 minutes per side.
- Add coconut milk mixture, water, and cod.
- Mix the soup gently and cook it with the closed lid for 20 minutes.

Lentils Soup

6 Servings

Preparation Time: 50 minutes

Ingredients

- 1 cup lentils
- 6 cups of water
- 1 onion, diced.
- 1 chili pepper, diced.
- 2 tbsps tomato paste
- 2 tbsps olive oil

Directions

- Mix onion with olive oil in the saucepan and roast for 2-3 minutes.
- Then add lentils, chili pepper, and tomato paste. Mix the mixture.
- Add water and mix the soup again.
- Close the lid and cook the soup for 25 minutes.

Mushroom Cream Soup

6 Servings

Preparation Time: 50 minutes

Ingredients

- 1-pound mushrooms, chopped.
- 1 cup plain yogurt
- 4 cups of water
- 2 onions, diced.
- 1 tablespoon olive oil
- 3 ounces Parmesan, grated.

Directions

- Mix olive oil with mushrooms in the saucepan and roast the mixture for 5 minutes.
- Add plain yogurt, water, onion, and simmer the soup for 20 minutes.
- Blend the soup with the help of the immersion blender and top with Parmesan.

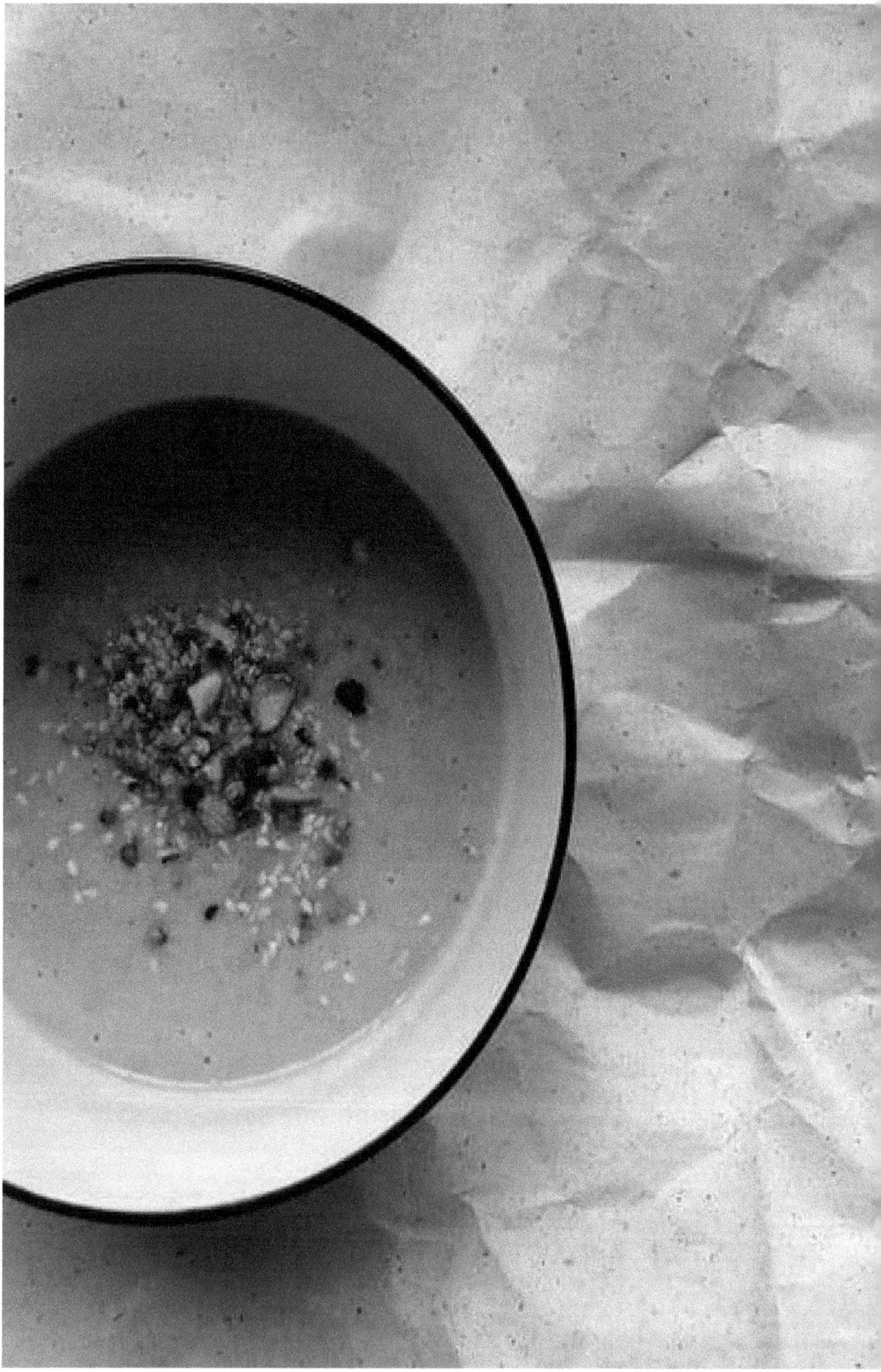

Meatball Soup

6 Servings

Preparation Time: 50 minutes

Ingredients

- 2 cups ground chicken
- 1 teaspoon chili powder
- 5 cups of water
- 1 onion, diced.
- 1 tablespoon olive oil
- 2 carrots, grated.

Directions

- Mix ground chicken with chili powder. Make the meatballs.
- Pour water in the saucepan.
- Add onion, olive oil, and carrot.
- Bring the soup to boil and add meatballs.
- Close the lid and cook the soup on medium heat for 20 minutes.

Tropical Soup

6 Servings

Preparation Time: 30 minutes

Ingredients

- 2 avocados, pitted. Peeled, chopped.
- 4 cups chicken stock
- 1 teaspoon lemongrass, chopped.
- 2 ounces chives, chopped.

Directions

- Bring the chicken stock to boil.
- Add lemongrass and chives.
- Then add avocados and remove the soup from heat.
- Let the soup rest for 5-10 minutes before serving.

DESSERTS

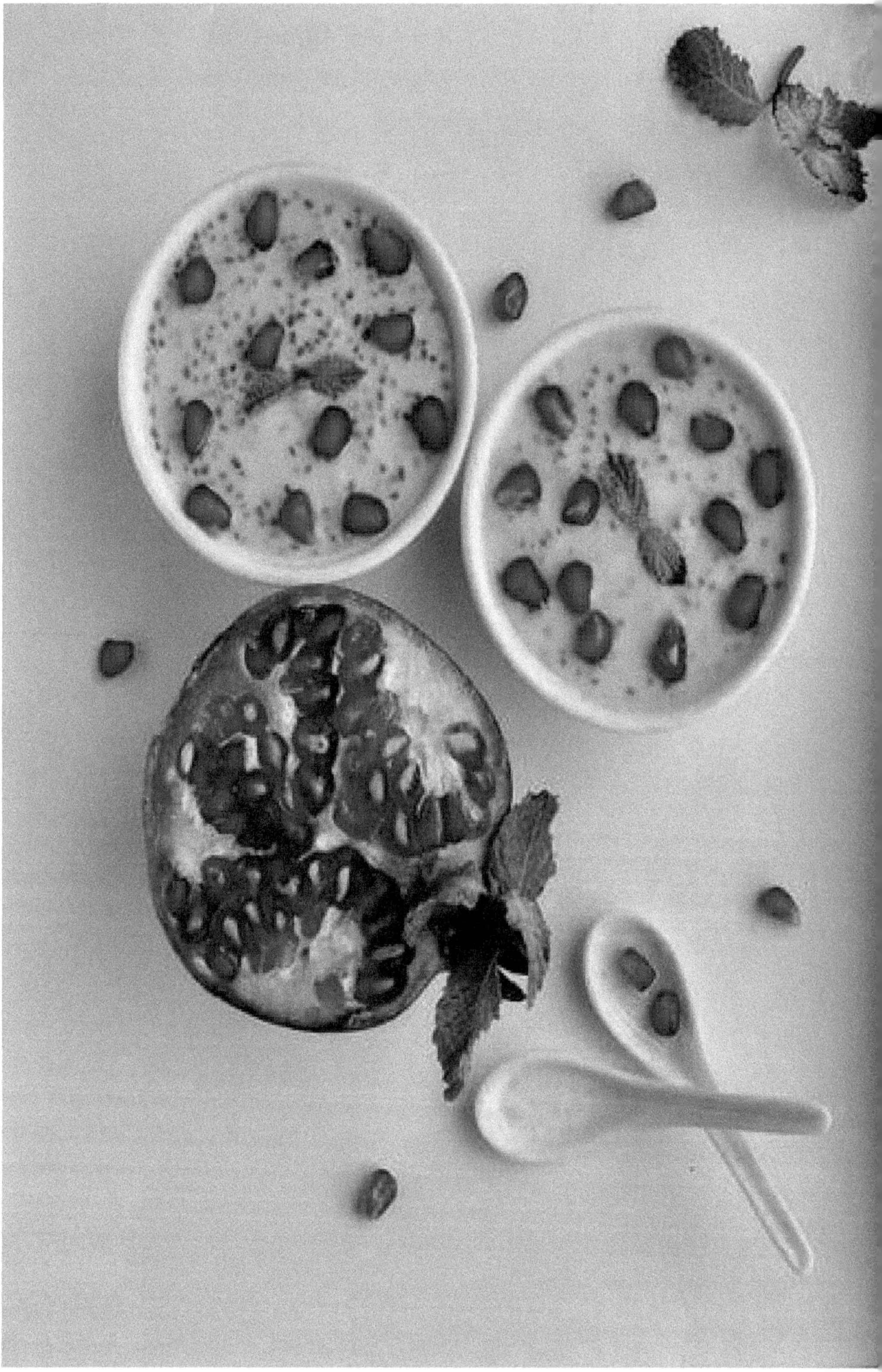

Pomegranate Bowls

6 Servings

Preparation Time: 2 hours and **30 minutes**

Ingredients

- Half cup coconut cream
- 1 orange, peeled and cut into wedges.
- 1 teaspoon vanilla extract
- Half cup almonds, chopped.
- 1 cup pomegranate seeds
- 1 tablespoon orange zest, grated.

Directions

- In a bowl, combine the orange with the pomegranate seeds and the other ingredients.
- Toss and keep in the fridge for 2 hours before dividing into smaller bowls and serving.

Maple Berries Bowls

6 Servings

Preparation Time: 20 minutes

Ingredients

- Half cup dates, pitted.
- Half teaspoon vanilla extract
- 1 cup almonds, chopped.
- 1 cup blackberries
- 1 tablespoon maple syrup
- 1 tablespoon coconut oil, melted.

Directions

- In a bowl, combine the berries with the almonds and the other ingredients.
- Toss, divide into small cups and serve.

Almond Rhubarb Pudding

8 Servings

Preparation Time: 40 minutes

Ingredients

- 2 cups rhubarb, sliced.
- 2 tbsps maple syrup
- 3 eggs
- 2 tbsps coconut oil, melted.
- 1 cup almond milk
- Half teaspoon baking powder

Directions

- In a blender, combine the rhubarb with the oil and maple syrup and pulse well.
- In a bowl, combine the rhubarb puree with the other ingredients.
- Whisk, divide into 6 ramekins and bake at 350 degrees F for 20 minutes.
- Serve the pudding cold.

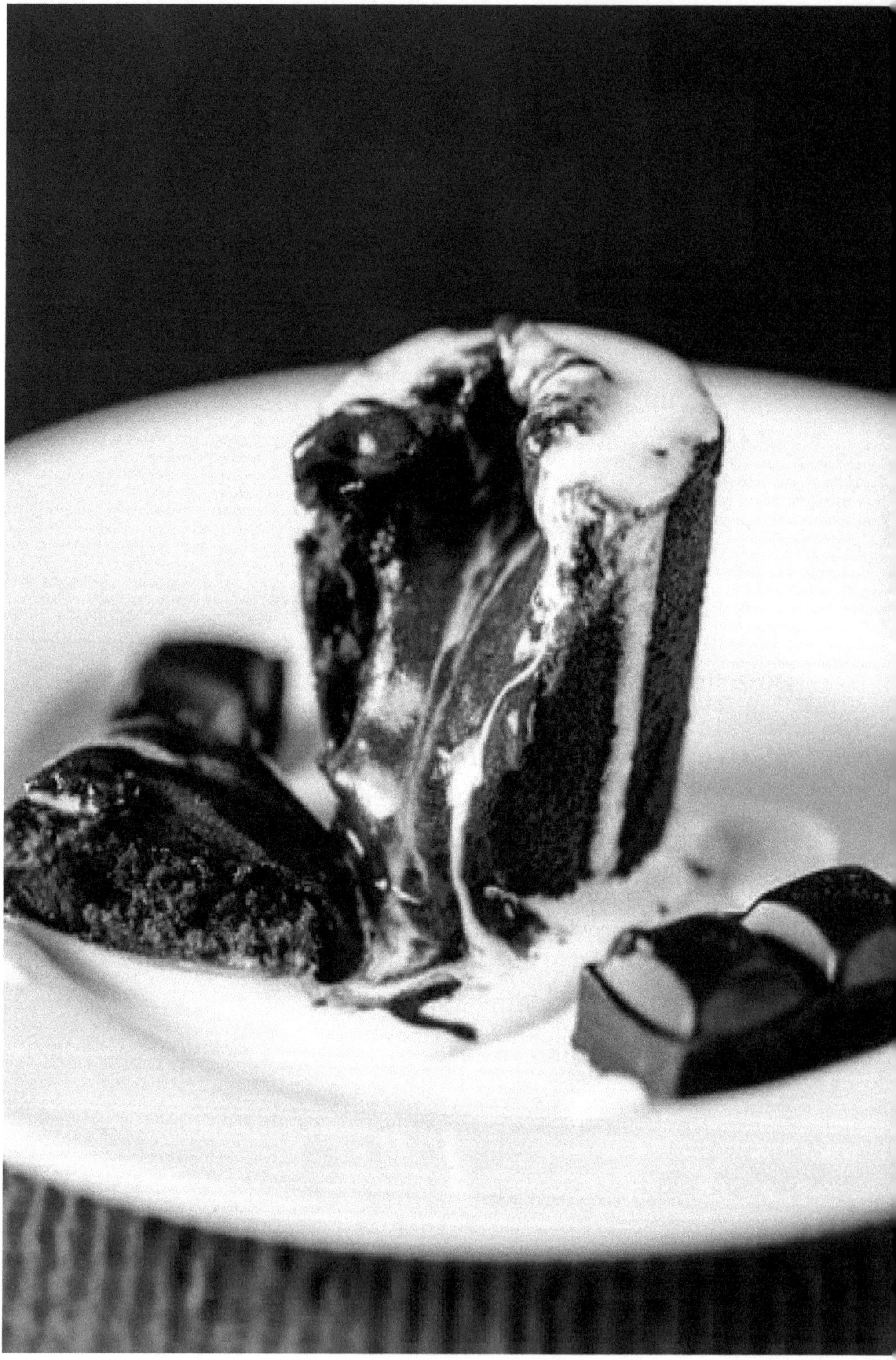

Dates and Pears Cake

8 Servings

Preparation Time: 50 minutes

Ingredients

- 2 pears, cored, peeled and chopped.
- 2 cups coconut flour
- 1 cup dates, pitted.
- 2 eggs, whisked.
- 1 teaspoon vanilla extract
- 1 teaspoon baking soda
- Half cup coconut oil, melted.
- Half teaspoon cinnamon powder

Directions

- In a bowl, combine the pears with the flour and the other ingredients.
- Whisk well, pour into a cake pan and bake at 360 degrees F for 30 minutes.
- Cool down, slice, and serve.

Pears Cream

6 Servings

Preparation Time: 20 minutes

Ingredients

- 2 teaspoons lime juice
- 1-pound pears, cored, peeled and chopped.
- 1-pound strawberries, chopped.
- 1 cup coconut cream

Directions

- In a blender, combine the pears with strawberries and the other ingredients, pulse well, divide into bowls and serve.

Orange Bowls

6 Servings

Preparation Time: 20 minutes

Ingredients

- 2 oranges peeled and cut into segments.
- 1 cantaloupe peeled and cubed.
- 2 tbsps honey
- 1 cup orange juice
- 1 teaspoon vanilla extract

Directions

- In a bowl, combine the oranges with the cantaloupe and the other ingredients.
- Toss and serve.

Chicory Cherry Cream

8 Servings

Preparation Time: 40 minutes

Ingredients

- 1-pound cherries, pitted. And chopped.
- Juice of 1 lime
- Zest of 1 lime, grated.
- 2 tbsps chicory root powder
- Quarter teaspoon vanilla extract

Directions

- In a pot, mix the cherries with the lime juice and the other ingredients, toss, and simmer over medium heat for 15 minutes.
- Blend using an immersion blender, divide into cups and serve cold.

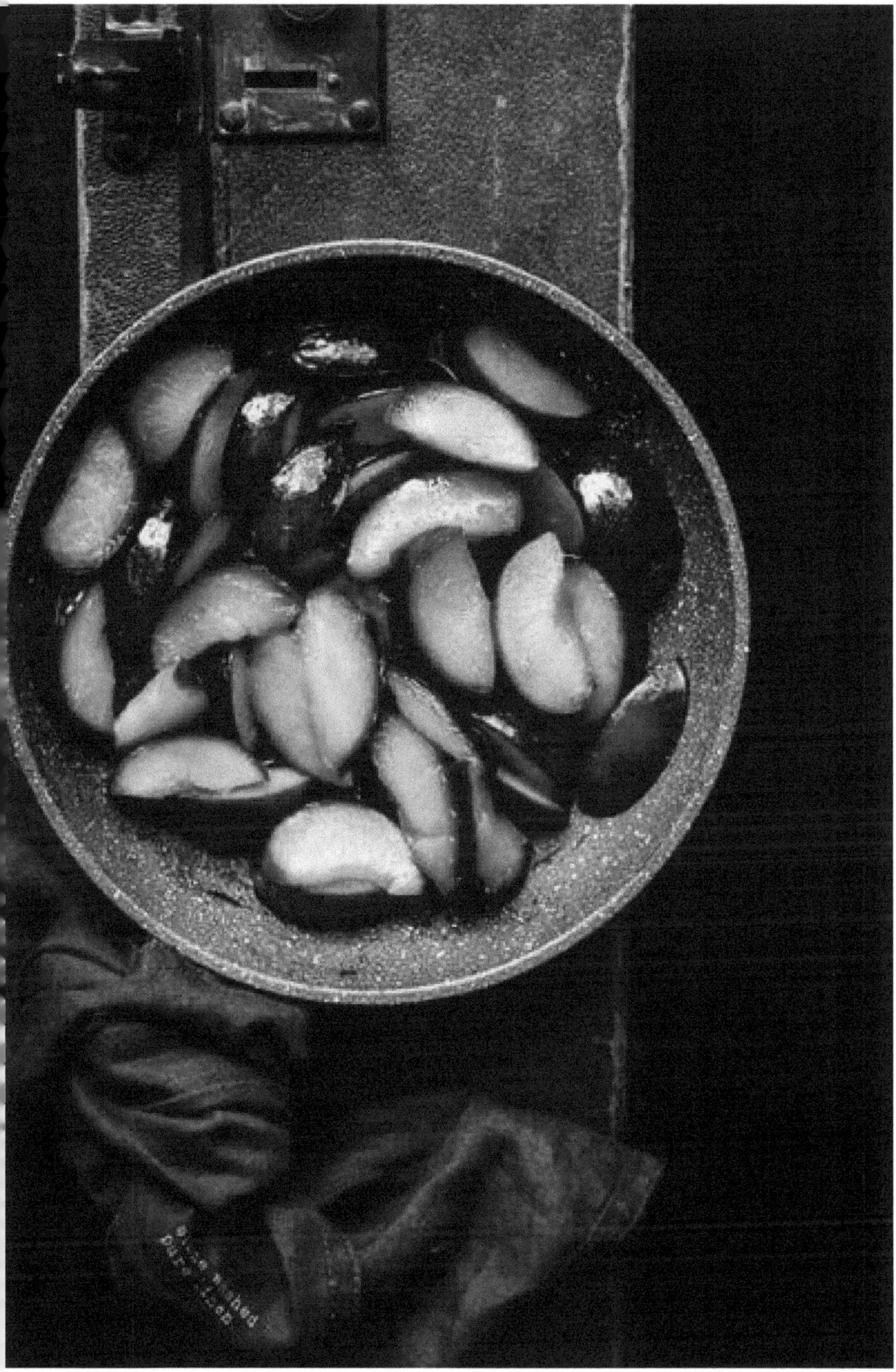

Cinnamon Apple Mix

8 Servings

Preparation Time: 40 minutes

Ingredients

- 3 apples cored and roughly cut into wedges.
- 3 pears cored and cut into wedges.
- 4 tbsps chicory root powder
- 2 teaspoons cinnamon powder

Directions

- In a roasting pan, combine the apples with the pears and the other ingredients, toss and cook at 380 degrees F for 20 minutes.
- Divide the mix between dessert plates and serve.

Lightning Source UK Ltd.
Milton Keynes UK
UKHW051148190521
383851UK00007B/73

9 781802 938517